BEYOND THE IMPACT

An Update on the Assessment, Prevention, and Treatment of Neuropsychiatric Sequelae Associated with Traumatic Brain Injury

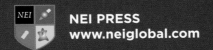

NEI PRESS
www.neiglobal.com

COPYRIGHT

PUBLISHED BY NEI PRESS, an imprint of NEUROSCIENCE EDUCATION INSTITUTE
Carlsbad, California, United States of America

NEUROSCIENCE EDUCATION INSTITUTE
5900 La Place Court, Suite 120
Carlsbad, California 92008

www.neiglobal.com

Printed in the United States of America
First Edition, August 2017
Electronic versions, August 2017

Typeset in Gotham

Library of Congress Cataloging-in-Publication Data
ISBN 1-4225-0056-X

Release / CME Expiration Dates

Print Monograph Released: August, 2017

Electronic Books Released: August, 2017

CME Credit Expires: August, 2020

Overview

Historically, the first major advancements in acute care of head injuries occurred after World War II, built on principles derived from military experiences and modern scientific, technological, and organizational progress. There has been a dramatic increase in civilian closed head injuries since the second half of the 20th century as a consequence of urbanization, roads, and the growing awareness of head injuries. In this book, we provide an update on the current knowledge of the neurobiological sequelae and genetic risk factors associated with traumatic brain injury (TBI). Next, we address the most current and effective screening tools to identify the occurrence and severity of symptoms associated with TBI. We also discuss neuropsychiatric conditions associated with TBI, and provide evidence-based guidance for accurate diagnosis and optimal treatment of TBI in high-risk populations.

Learning Objectives

After completing this activity, you should be better able to:

- Identify neurobiological and genetic substrates associated with neuropsychiatric sequelae of TBI

- Update knowledge on recent advances in the prevention of neuropsychiatric complications following TBI

- Provide a differential diagnosis of psychiatric conditions following TBI

- Utilize appropriate treatment strategies for patients with TBI and comorbid neuropsychiatric disorders

Optional Posttest and CME Credit Instructions

There is no posttest fee nor fee for CME credits. The estimated time for completion of this activity is 6.0 hours.

1. Read the book

2. Complete the posttest, only online, at **www.neiglobal.com/CME** (under "Book")

3. Print your certificate (if a score of 70% or more is achieved)

Questions? call 888-535-5600, or email **CustomerService@NEIglobal.com**

Accreditation and Credit Designation Statements

The Neuroscience Education Institute is accredited by the Accreditation Council for Continuing Medical Education (ACCME) to provide continuing medical education for physicians.

The Neuroscience Education Institute designates this enduring material for a maximum of 6.0 *AMA PRA Category 1 Credits*™. Physicians should claim only the credit commensurate with the extent of their participation in the activity.

The American Society for the Advancement of Pharmacotherapy (ASAP), Division 55 of the American Psychological Association, is approved by the American Psychological Association to sponsor continuing education for psychologists. ASAP maintains responsibility for this program and its content.

The American Society for the Advancement of Pharmacotherapy designates this program for 6.0 CE credits for psychologists.

Nurses and **Physician Assistants:** for your CE requirements, the ANCC and NCCPA will accept *AMA PRA Category 1 Credits*™ from organizations accredited by the AMA (providers accredited by the ACCME). A portion of the content in this activity pertains to pharmacology and is worth 2.0 continuing education hours of pharmacotherapeutics.

A certificate of participation for completing this activity is available.

Note: the content of this print monograph activity also exists as an electronic book under the same title. If you received CME credit for the electronic book version, you will not be able to receive credit again for completing this print monograph version.

Peer Review

This material has been peer-reviewed by an MD specializing in psychiatry to ensure the scientific accuracy and medical relevance of information presented and its independence from commercial bias. NEI takes responsibility for the content, quality, and scientific integrity of this CME activity.

Disclosures

All individuals in a position to influence or control content are required to disclose any financial relationships. Although potential conflicts of interest are identified and resolved prior to the activity being presented, it remains for the participant to determine whether outside interests reflect a possible bias in either the exposition or the conclusions presented.

Disclosed financial relationships with conflicts of interest have been reviewed by the NEI CME Advisory Board Chair and resolved.

Author / Developer

Sabrina Kay Segal, PhD
Adjunct Professor, Department of Psychology, Arizona State University, Tempe, AZ
Adjunct Professor, Biological Sciences, Palomar College, San Marcos, CA
Medical Writer, Neuroscience Education Institute, Carlsbad, CA
No financial relationships to disclose.

Content Editor

Stephen M. Stahl, MD, PhD
Adjunct Professor, Department of Psychiatry, University of California, San Diego School of Medicine, La Jolla, CA
Honorary Visiting Senior Fellow, University of Cambridge, Cambridge, UK
Director of Psychopharmacology, California Department of State Hospitals, Sacramento, CA
Grant/Research: Acadia, Avanir, Braeburn, Intra-Cellular, Ironshore, Lilly, Neurocrine, Otsuka, Shire, Sunovion
Consultant/Advisor: Acadia, Alkermes, Allergan, Arbor, AstraZeneca, Axovant, Biogen, Biopharma, Celgene, Forest, Forum, Genomind, Innovative Science Solutions, Intra-Cellular, Jazz, Lundbeck, Merck, Otsuka, Pamlab, Servier, Shire, Sunovion, Takeda, Teva
Speakers Bureau: Forum, Lundbeck, Otsuka, Perriog, Servier, Sunovion, Takeda
Board Member: Genomind

Peer Reviewer

William M. Sauvé, MD
Medical Director, Greenbrook TMS NeuroHealth Centers of Richmond and Charlottesville, Glen Allen and Charlottesville, VA
Speakers Bureau: Avanir, Otsuka, Sunovion

The **Design Staff** has no financial relationships to disclose.

CME INFORMATION

Disclosure of Off-Label Use

This educational activity may include discussion of unlabeled and/or investigational uses of agents that are not currently labeled for such use by the FDA. Please consult the product prescribing information for full disclosure of labeled uses.

Disclaimer

Participants have an implied responsibility to use the newly acquired information from this activity to enhance patient outcomes and their own professional development. The information presented in this educational activity is not meant to serve as a guideline for patient management. Any procedures, medications, or other courses of diagnosis or treatment discussed or suggested in this educational activity should not be used by clinicians without evaluation of their patients' conditions and possible contraindications or dangers in use, review of any applicable manufacturer's product information, and comparison with recommendations of other authorities. Primary references and full prescribing information should be consulted.

Cultural and Linguistic Competency

A variety of resources addressing cultural and linguistic competency can be found at this link: **nei.global/CMEregs**

Provider

This activity is provided by NEI.
Additionally provided by the American Society for the Advancement of Pharmacotherapy.

Support

This activity is supported by an unrestricted educational grant from Avanir Pharmaceuticals, Inc.

OBJECTIVES

- Identify neurobiological and genetic substrates associated with neuropsychiatric sequelae of TBI

- Update knowledge on recent advances in the prevention of neuropsychiatric complications following TBI

- Provide a differential diagnosis of psychiatric conditions following TBI

- Utilize appropriate treatment strategies for patients with TBI and comorbid neuropsychiatric disorders

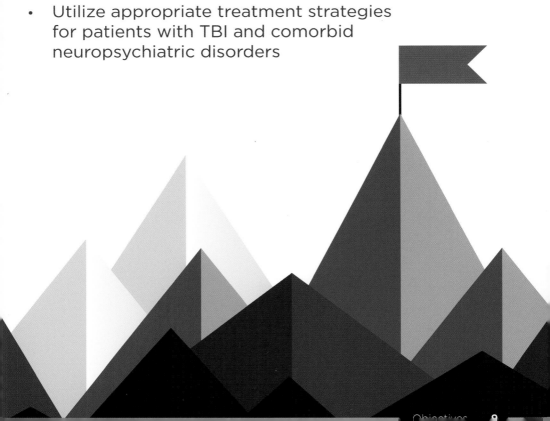

INTRODUCTION

Historically, the first major advancements in acute care of head injuries occurred after World War II, built on principles derived from military experiences, and modern scientific, technological, and organizational progress. There has been a dramatic increase in civilian closed head injuries since the second half of the 20th century, as a consequence of urbanization, roads, and the growing awareness of head injuries. In this book, we provide an update on the current knowledge of the neurobiological sequelae and genetic risk factors associated with traumatic brain injury (TBI). Next, we address the most current and effective screening tools to identify the occurrence and severity of symptoms associated with TBI. We also discuss neuropsychiatric conditions associated with TBI, and provide evidence-based guidance for accurate diagnosis and optimal treatment of TBI in high-risk populations.

CHAPTER 1

Neurobiological Sequelae and Genetic Risk Factors Associated with Traumatic Brain Injury

In Chapter 1, we address the epidemiology of traumatic brain injuries (TBIs), and the neurological damage that can occur from various types of head trauma. We present the most common types of head injuries/neurological damage from specific high risk populations for TBIs, namely military personnel, athletes, and victims of physical violence/abuse. In this chapter, we also address genetic risk factors and neurobiological sequelae associated with TBI. Finally, we address age-specific neurobiological consequences of multiple TBIs, such as Second Impact Syndrome (SIS) in adolescents and chronic traumatic encephalopathy (CTE) in adults.

TRAUMATIC BRAIN INJURY (TBI)

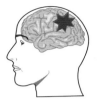

Glasgow Coma Scale (GCS)	Cantu Grading Scale
Score of 13-15: Mild Traumatic Brain Injury	Grade 1 (mild) No loss of consciousness; Post-traumatic amnesia* or post-concussion signs or symptoms lasting less than 30 minutes
Score of 9-12 Moderate Traumatic Brain Injury	Grade 2 (moderate) Loss of consciousness lasting less than 1 minute; Post-traumatic amnesia* or post-concussion signs or symptoms lasting longer than 30 minutes but less than 24 hours
Score of ≤ 8 Severe Traumatic Brain Injury	Grade 3 (severe) Loss of consciousness lasting more than 1 minute; Post-traumatic amnesia* lasting longer than 24 hours; Post-concussion signs or symptoms lasting longer than 7 days

FIGURE 1.1.

According to the Brain Injury Association of America (BIAA), "TBI is defined as an alteration in brain function, or other evidence of brain pathology, caused by an external force." The Glasgow Coma Scale (GCS; Teasdale & Jennett, 1974) is the measurement tool most frequently used to measure the level of consciousness immediately following an injury. The GCS score is based on a 15-point behavioral observation scale, which grades behavioral responses into three categories (i.e., eye opening, motor response, and verbal response). A GCS score of 8 or less indicates a severe TBI, a score of 9–12 places an individual in the moderate severity group, and a score of 13–15 indicates a mild TBI (mTBI). The score is thought to reflect the structural and functional status of the central nervous system immediately following injury. A grading scale for the severity of TBI, based on the presence of amnesia, was developed by Cantu in 1986). *Retrograde and anterograde

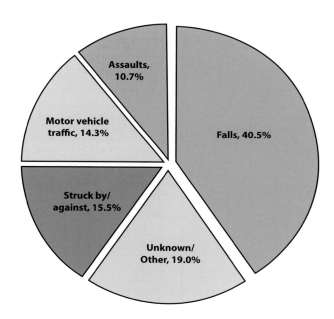

FIGURE 1.2.

According to the Center for Disease Control (CDC), there are approximately 2.5 million emergency department (ED) visits, hospitalizations, or deaths associated with TBI in the United States. There are many more that go unreported. According to the CDC, from 2006-2010 the leading cause of TBI associated with ED visits was falls. 55% of TBIs among children 0 to 14 years were caused by falls. 81% of TBIs in adults aged 65 and older are caused by falls. Unintentional blunt trauma was the second leading cause of ER-related TBI, accounting for about 15% of TBIs in the United States. Close to 24% of all TBIs in children less than 15 years of age were related to blunt trauma. Among all age groups, motor vehicle crashes were the third overall leading cause of TBI-related deaths. About 10% of ER-related TBIs are due to assaults. Approximately 75% of all assaults associated with TBI occur in people 15 to 44 years of age. Since 2001, over 1.5 million American military personnel have served and an alarming rate of 22% of all wounded soldiers have suffered a TBI (Okie et al., 2005). An estimated 1.6-3.8 million sports-related TBIs occur annually. Of these, only 300,000 result in loss of consciousness (LOC) (Langlois et al., 2006).

NEUROPATHOLOGICAL CONSEQUENCES OF DIFFERENT TRAUMATIC BRAIN INJURY TYPES

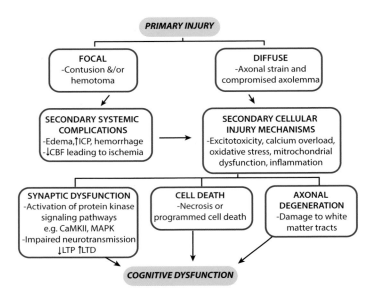

FIGURE 1.3.

While there are a variety of types of injuries that can result in traumatic brain injury (TBI) (e.g. blunt force, strangling, blast explosion), there are two main phases of injury that can result in cognitive dysfunction. The primary injury (direct impact or rotational/acceleration) results in focal or diffuse injury. While these types of injuries differ in neurophysiological responses, they each give rise to secondary systemic complications and cellular injury mechanisms that result in cell death, axonal injury, and impaired synaptic plasticity. The extent of cell death and axonal injury correlates strongly with neurological outcome following TBI. In the case of mild TBI (mTBI), while no overt cell loss is detected, chronic cognitive deficits may be observed. This is likely due to impairments in synaptic plasticity that contribute to cognitive dysfunction (Walker et al., 2013). ICP = intracranial pressure, CBF = cerebral blood flow, CaMKII = Calmodulin-Dependent Protein Kinase II, MAPK = microtubule-associated protein kinase, LTP = long-term potentiation, LTD = long-term depression.

SIGNS AND SYMPTOMS OF TRAUMATIC BRAIN INJURY

Physical

Cognitive

Emotional

insomnia

Sleep

Postconcussion Syndrome (PCS)

Headaches

Dizziness

Short-term memory problems

Noise sensitivity

Light sensitivity

FIGURE 1.4.

The signs and symptoms of concussion fall into 4 categories: physical, cognitive, emotional, and sleep (CDC, 2012). Headache is the most common symptom, with frequency between 40% and 86% (Fazio et al., 2007). Postconcussion syndrome (PCS) is defined as the persistence of post-concussive symptoms beyond the expected time frame of 1 to 6 weeks (Jotwani et al., 2010). The incidence is estimated to be approximately 10% (Prigatano et al., 2011). Postconcussion syndrome is a complex disorder with symptoms occurring 7 to 10 days after a mild traumatic brain injury (mTBI), lasting for weeks to months, and up to a year or more in some individuals. The constellation of symptoms includes headache, dizziness, fatigue, difficulty concentrating, irritability, anxiety, and noise and light sensitivity. The severity of the injury does not correlate with the duration or type of symptoms. Persons experiencing PCS report limitations in functional status, activities of daily living, school- or work-related activities, leisure and recreational activities, social interactions, and financial independence. (Silverberg et al., 2011). Risk factors include: comorbid psychiatric illness, advanced age, heightened symptoms, and intense emotions, such as severe anxiety at the time of injury (Prigatano et al., 2011).

	Type of Injury	Neurological Damage
	Blow to the head with an object	Damage to underlying tissue/vessels
	Thrown against a wall or solid surface	Focal and diffuse damage
	Punched in the face or head	Contusions, bruising/bleeding
	Violent shaking of the body	Diffuse axonal injuries/torn nerve tissue
	Falling and hitting your head	Focal and diffuse damage
	Being strangled	Diffuse damage (hypoxia)
	Near drowning	Diffuse damage (hypoxia)
	Being shot in the face or head	Disintegration of brain tissue

FIGURE 1.5.

The most common head injuries that occur in high-risk populations for traumatic brain injuries (TBIs) differ, depending on the environment, resulting in various types of neurological damage. In military combat personnel, the most common head injury is mild traumatic brain injury (mTBI), induced by high pressure changes during a blast explosion (Michael et al., 2015), typically resulting in diffuse axonal damage. For athletes, the most common type of head injuries occur from direct blunt force (being hit in the head or neck region), or rotational acceleration/deacceleration injuries, resulting in focal and diffuse damage. Victims of interpersonal violence (IPV) may experience a broad range of head injuries (from direct blunt force to strangulation), which may result in focal injuries, such as torn nerve tissue, along with diffuse injuries, such as hypoxia. Ultimately, all head injuries have the potential to result in neuron death (Iverson et al., 2017).

CHRONIC TRAUMATIC ENCEPHALOPATHY (CTE) NEUROPATHOLOGY

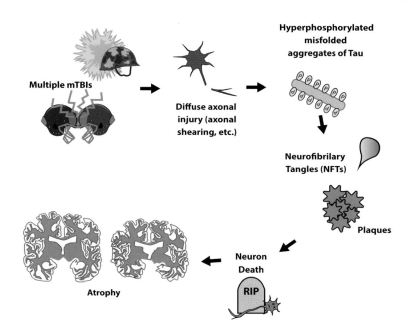

FIGURE 1.6.

Chronic Traumatic Encephalopathy (CTE) is a progressive degenerative disease that results from repetitive head trauma. At least 17% of patients who experience repeated mTBIs develop CTE (McKee et al., 2009). The proposed underlying mechanism is diffuse axonal injury, which leads to neurofibrillary tangles (NFTs) in the frontal and temporal cortices. The NFTs are caused by misfolded aggregates of tau protein that result in tau prions. In CTE postmortem studies, approximately 50% of brains with NFTs also have diffuse Aβ plaques (DeKosky et al., 2013). Postmortem studies report atrophy of cerebral hemispheres, medial temporal lobe, thalamus, mammillary bodies, and brain stem, with ventricular dilation and fenestrated cavum septum pellucidum. In CTE, the NFTs are found in more superficial cortical layers, whereas in Alzheimer's disease (AD), the NFTs are observed in deeper cortical layers. CTE was first identified in American National Football League (NFL) players, yet the neuropathology is indistinguishable from dementia pugilistica, detected in boxers years prior to the identification of CTE (DeKosky et al., 2013). In a recent postmortem study, 96% of NFL players' brains had tau pathology, characteristic of CTE. Only a handful of studies have examined CTE in military veterans. A recent study found evidence of classic CTE tau pathology in the brains of 4 military veterans who were exposed to multiple blasts, or a single close-range blast (McKee et al., 2013). There have been no studies to date on the incidence of CTE in victims of IPV.

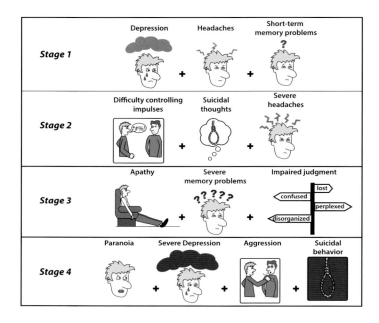

FIGURE 1.7.

Symptoms arise from four stages of CTE. In Stage 1, patients may experience depression, headaches, and short-term memory loss. In Stage 2, they may have difficulty controlling impulses, or suicidal thoughts, and have severe headaches. Stage 3 is typically characterized by apathy, severe memory problems, and impaired judgment. In Stage 4 patients may experience paranoia, severe depression, aggression, dementia, and suicidal behaviors (McKee et al., 2013).

HIGH RISK POPULATION FOR ADULT TRAUMATIC BRAIN INJURY: ATHLETES

History of Concussion Awareness in the National Football League (NFL)

Dr. Omalu's findings published in the journal "Neurosurgery"

2005

NFL holds its first concussions summit

2007

2002

Steelers Hall of Fame football player, Mike Webster, dies at age 50. Dr. Bennet Omalu examines his brain at autopsy and identifies disease pathology as CTE.

2006

Former Eagles football player Andre Waters commits suicide with gunshot to head

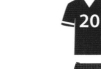

2009

NFL-funded study reveals former players have cognitive impairment

FIGURE 1.8.

One of the highest at-risk populations for mild traumatic brain injury (mTBI) and Chronic Traumatic Encephalopathy (CTE) are professional American football players in the National Football League (NFL). However, for years, the NFL was resistant to recognizing or researching the detrimental effects of football on the brain. The past fifteen years of research on this high-risk population has offered several useful findings on both mTBI in athletes and CTE in this high-risk population. For athletes in high-contact sports, the most common head injury is mTBI resulting from a blow to the head or acceleration-deceleration. This type of injury can severely impact axonal projections and small blood vessels within and from the brain stem, in the parasagittal white matter of the cerebrum, corpus callosum, and gray-white junctions of the cerebral cortex, and the gray-white junctions in the ventral, anterior, frontal, and temporal lobes (McAllister et al., 2011). Up to 15% of patients who experience mTBI will develop persistent cognitive dysfunction. At least 17% of patients who experience repeated mTBIs develop CTE (McKee et al., 2009).

History of Concussion Awareness in the National Football League (NFL)

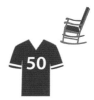

First series of lawsuits filed by former players against the NFL	Former San Diego Chargers Junior Seau commits suicide. Autopsy reveals CTE	NFL announces new safety measures, neurologist on sideline for games	49ers Chris Borland abruptly retires from football, after TBI
2011	**2012**	**2013**	**2015**

2011
Former Chicago Bear Dave Duerson commits suicide with gunshot to chest. Autopsy reveals CTE.

2012
NFL funds "Heads Up Football" to raise safety awareness in youth.

2013
"A League of Denial" is published, exposing the NFL crisis

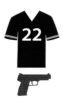

FIGURE 1.8. continued

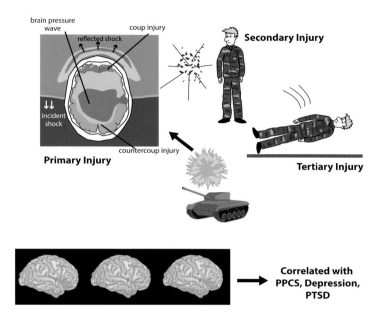

FIGURE 1.9.

The most common form of head injury in the military today is blast-induced mild traumatic brain injury (mTBI). Detonation of explosive devices results in a pressure wave, inducing a sudden increase in intracranial pressure and resulting in penetration of brain tissue, disruption of axonal pathways, and damage to capillaries (Magnuson et al., 2012). These blast-induced effects are referred to as primary injury. The blast wave may also propel objects toward a person causing secondary injury, or it may force the person into other solid objects/surfaces, referred to as tertiary injury. While secondary and tertiary injuries are consistent with contact-induced TBI, primary injury is generally unique to blast events and may have independent consequences on brain tissue structure and function. Recent research suggests that mild and moderate blast-induced TBIs result in cortical thinning in the right insula and inferior temporal and frontal lobes for 5 months to 10 years after TBI (Michael et al., 2015). Cortical thickness values correlated with measures of PTSD, depression, and post-concussive symptoms (Michael et al., 2015). Blast-induced mTBI typically appears normal on conventional neuroimaging scans, such as Magnetic Resonance Imaging (MRI) or Computed Tomography (CT), however, over 50% of veterans meet criteria for post-concussive disorder at long-term follow-up post injury. PPCS = Persistent Post Concussive Symptoms, PTSD = Post Traumatic Stress Disorder.

TRAUMATIC BRAIN INJURY IN ADOLESCENTS

Causes of TBIs in Adolescents According to Frequency:

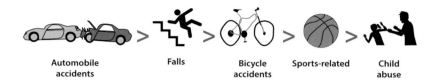

Automobile accidents > Falls > Bicycle accidents > Sports-related > Child abuse

Effects of TBIs on Behavioral/Social Problems in Adolescents

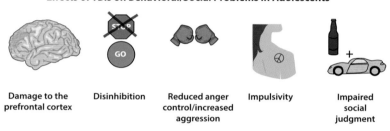

Damage to the prefrontal cortex | Disinhibition | Reduced anger control/increased aggression | Impulsivity | Impaired social judgment

FIGURE 1.10.

TBI is the leading cause of death in children and adolescents, according the Center for Disease Control and Prevention (CDC). According to the CDC, automobile accidents account for the highest frequency of TBIs in this population, while assault accounts for the lowest frequency. The two age groups at highest risk are 0-4 and 15-19. Brain injury will typically have more devastating consequences on a developing brain, such as a child or adolescent. Fletcher et al. (1996) reported postinjury problems in approximately 30% of children/adolescents with severe brain injury. In the early weeks and months after a severe brain injury, challenging behaviors may be a direct result of the injury. Damage to the prefrontal areas of the brain, the most common site of lesion in closed head injury (Levin et al., 1991), can result in disinhibition, impulsiveness, reduced anger control, aggressiveness, and poor social judgment (Stuss and Benson, 1987; Varney and Menefee, 1993).

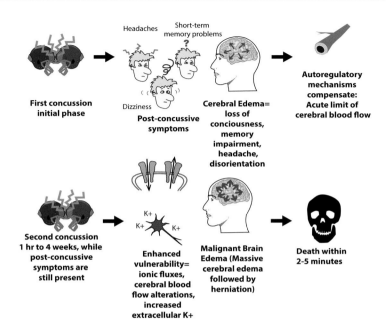

FIGURE 1.11.

Second Impact Syndrome (SIS), first described in 1984 (Saunders and Harbaugh, 1984), consists of two events. First, it involves an athlete suffering from post-concussive symptoms following a traumatic brain injury (TBI) (Cantu et al., 1998). If the athlete returns to play too soon and sustains a second TBI, diffuse cerebral swelling, brain herniation, and even death can occur within minutes. A patient who sustains an initial concussion may develop cerebral edema, accounting for loss of consciousness (LOC) and postconcussive symptoms. The brain's autoregulatory mechanisms compensate for this mechanical and physiological stress and protect against massive swelling. However, extracellular potassium concentration can increase massively after concussion, making the brain more vulnerable and susceptible to death after a second sublethal insult of even less intensity (Maroon et al., 2000). While rare, SIS may have devastating consequences, particularly for adolescents (Bey and Ostick, 2008). The existence of SIS is widely debated throughout the literature. There is controversy surrounding (1) whether the edema in SIS is truly due to a second hit or whether it is progression of injury from a single hit; (2) how far apart the first and second hits can be; (3) whether subdural hematomas or other structural anomalies play a significant role in the progression to severe edema; and (4) why far more cases are reported in the United States than elsewhere (McLendon et al., 2016).

TRAUMATIC BRAIN INJURY IN INFANTS AND YOUNG CHILDREN

Etiology of TBIs in children 0-3 years old

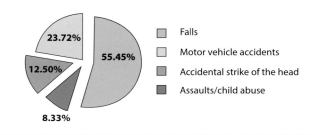

- Falls
- Motor vehicle accidents
- Accidental strike of the head
- Assaults/child abuse

Structural Considerations that Result in Different Types of TBIs in Infants Compared to Adults

 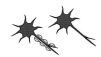

Infant brain is smaller and lighter than the adult brain

Undeveloped myelin sheaths in many regions of the infant brain

Undeveloped neck muscle and poor head support. Vertebral body is prone to dislocation

FIGURE 1.12.

Falls account for the highest incidence of traumatic brain injury (TBI) in young children and infants, followed by motor vehicle accidents, being accidentally hit on the head, and child abuse (Ciurea et al., 2011). Recent research findings suggest that the development of infants and young children may be more adversely affected by brain injury than the development of older children and adolescents (Eslinger et al., 2004). Structurally, there are unique biomechanical properties for pediatric brain injury due to a combination of higher plasticity and deformity, whereby external forces are absorbed in a different way compared to adults. While the infant and toddler brain is smaller/lighter than the adult brain, it is heavier compared to their body, thus the likelihood of head trauma is higher. In addition, temporal differences between myelination of various brain areas are pronounced during progressing development, and there are fewer myelinated axons than in the adult brain, leading to increased susceptibility to TBI in the unmyelinated regions (Araki et al., 2017). Finally, young children have weaker neck muscles, and the head is relatively heavy, thus the vertebral body is prone to dislocation (Araki et al., 2017).

Acute signs of concussion

Vomiting

Headache

Crying/Inability to Console

Restlessness/ Irritability

Persistent signs of concussion

Excessive crying

Persistent headache

Poor attention

Change in sleep patterns

FIGURE 1.13.

Young children may have the same concussion symptoms as older children, but they do not express them in the same way. For example, young children cannot explain a feeling of nausea or amnesia or even describe where they hurt. The most common acute signs of concussion in infants/young children are: vomiting, headache, crying/inability to console, and restlessness or irritability. Children who are suspected of having a concussion should be seen by a primary care physician (PCP). If persistent signs emerge, they should be seen by a neurologist, neuropsychologist, or other specialist. The most common persistent signs of concussion in infants/young children are: excessive crying, persistent headache, poor attention, and change in sleep patterns (Brain Injury Association of America, 2017).

TRAUMATIC BRAIN INJURY IN INFANTS AND YOUNG CHILDREN

PRIMARY INJURIES

Injury Type	Injury Cause	Neuropathology
Skull Fracture (Depressed, Basal, Ping-Pong)	Localized external force	Basal fracture: cranial nerve and vascular injuries
Acute Epidural Hematoma	Birth-related head injury in neonates	Cerebral herniation, even death
Acute Subdural Hematoma	Rupture caused by direct external force or collision of a moving skull with a stationary object	Vascular and cerebral parenchymal injury
Subdural Fluid Accumulation	Abusive Head Trauma	Can vary from hematoma to high protein concentration
Traumatic Subarachnoid Hemorrhage (tSAH)	Microvascular ruptures in subarachnoid pace or on the brain surface	Indicative of TBI severity in pediatric patients
Intraventricular hemorrhage (IVH)	Intraventricular perforations of intracerebral hematomas located next to the cerebral ventricles	Post-traumatic hydrocephalus
Cerebral Contusions	Lesions that occur just below the site of impact of external force (coup injury)	Cerebral swelling may develop into extensive hypoxic lesion
Diffuse Axonal Injury (DAI)	Blood vessels and nerve fibers are injured by shear force	Changes in white matter in the frontal and parietal lobes, auditory ampulla, basal ganglia, internal capsule, and corpus callosum

SECONDARY INJURIES

Injury Type	Injury Cause	Neuropathology
Diffuse Cerebral Swelling	Most commonly associated with Abusive Head Trauma	Cerebral hyperemia which can result in serious intracranial hypertension

FIGURE 1.14.

(Araki et al., 2017)

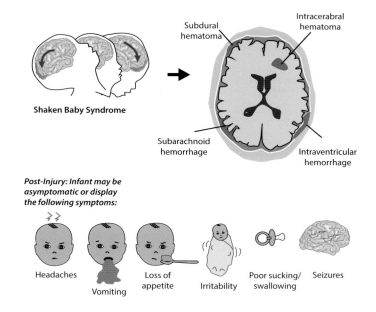

FIGURE 1.15.

Abusive Head Trauma (AHT), or Shaken Baby Syndrome, is the leading cause of severe brain injury and death in children less than 2 years old (Chiesa and Duhaime, Pediatric Clin North Am, 2009; Parks, Kegler, Annest, InjPrev, 2011). Children younger than 5 years account for 81.5% of all child abuse, with those younger than 1 year being the most vulnerable group. Primary injuries are caused by direct impact from the head trauma and involve retinal hemorrhages, skull fractures, intracranial hemorrhages, parenchymal injuries, and spinal cord injuries, whereas secondary injuries typically involve hypoxia or ischemia. The most common characteristic of AHT is intracranial hemorrhage (ICH), which can be divided into subdural hemorrhage, epidural hemorrhage, or subarachnoid hemorrhage. After AHT, children can be asymptomatic, or have lethargy, irritability, decreased appetite, poor sucking or swallowing, nausea, emesis, headache, or seizures (Kim and Falcone, 2017).

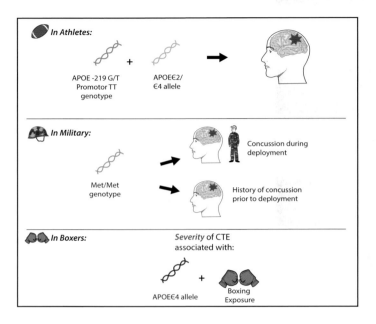

FIGURE 1.16.

A recent systematic review examined the association between genetics and risk for sustaining a traumatic brain injury (TBI). An association was found between those who carry a APOE-e2/e4 allele in addition to the T allele of -219 G/T. United States soldiers with the Met/Met genotype for Brain Derived Neurotrophic Factor (BDNF) were more likely to report a history of concussion prior to deployment and to sustain a concussion during deployment. Recent research found that the APOEε4 allele was present in 38% of 45 retired National Football League (NFL) players (Casson et al., 2014). The pathology for chronic traumatic encephalopathy (CTE) is indistinguishable from dementia pugilistica, thus it is referred to here as CTE in boxers. In boxers, the severity of CTE has been associated with the presence of the APOEε4 allele and the extent of boxing exposure. In addition, when a cohort of boxers was compared to controls, 50% of boxers carried the APOEε4 allele, compared to 11% of controls (DeKosky et al., 2013).

CHAPTER 2

Screening for the Occurrence, Severity, Symptoms, and Environmental Risk Factors Associated with Traumatic Brain Injury

In Chapter 2, we present the most current, valid screening methods for the detection of traumatic brain injury (TBI), especially in high-risk populations. We discuss the most sensitive neuroimaging techniques for the detection of a variety of TBI types (e.g., blast-induced versus blunt force), and for the detection of Chronic Traumatic Encephalopathy (CTE). We also present biomarkers associated with neurological damage, as well as post-concussive symptoms and cognitive symptoms that often accompany TBI. Finally, we address environmental risk factors predictive of TBI in adolescents, and signs that may be indicative of abusive head trauma in infants.

Chapter 2: Screening for the Occurrence, Severity, Symptoms, and Environmental Risk Factors Associated with Traumatic Brain Injury

31

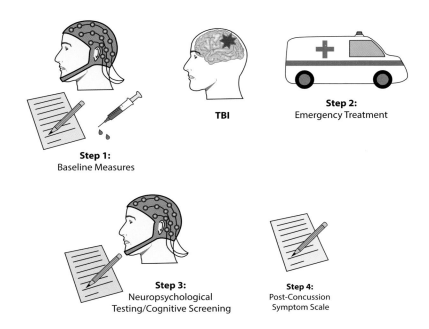

Step 1:
Baseline Measures

TBI

Step 2:
Emergency Treatment

Step 3:
Neuropsychological
Testing/Cognitive Screening

Step 4:
Post-Concussion
Symptom Scale

FIGURE 2.1.

For high-risk populations (athletes, military, and victims of intimate partner violence) patients will benefit tremendously if the following steps are taken in detecting traumatic brain injury (TBI). Step 1: Baseline Testing in the form of biological biomarkers, neuroimaging, and/or neuropsychological tests. Step 2: Emergency medical treatment immediately following TBI. Step 3: Neuropsychological testing and standardized cognitive screening immediately following emergency medical treatment. Step 4: Post-concussive symptom follow-up with standardized measures, such as the Post-Concussion Symptom Scale (PCSS).

ATHLETES

Sideline Screening Assessment	Evaluates
Immediate Post-Concussive Assessment and Cognitive Testing (ImPACT)	Immediate and delayed memory for words; immediate and delayed memory for designs, attention, concentration, working memory, reaction speed, response inhibition, visual-motor speed
Sports Concussion Assessment Tool (SCAT)	Loss of consciousness, signs, memory, symptoms, cognitive assessment, neurologic screening
Standardized Assessment of Concussion (SAC)	Orientation, immediate memory, neurological screening, concentration, exertional maneuvers, delayed memory recall
Acute Concussion Evaluation (ACE)	Injury characteristics, symptom checklist (physical, cognitive, emotional, sleep), concussion history/risk factors, red flags for reference to emergency department, diagnosis, and follow-up plan
King-Devick Test in association with Mayo Clinic	Saccadic eye movements using Rapid Number Naming (RNN™) to help determine neurological functionality with 90% accuracy in diagnosing concussion

FIGURE 2.2.

Broglio et al. (2007) found that a complete battery of tests, including assessment of neurocognitive functioning, self-reported symptom assessments, and postural control evaluation, was more sensitive to concussions than was each test individually. These are the most current, validated screening tools developed for immediate assessment of TBI in athletes on the sidelines. While ImPACT is the only FDA-approved concussion assessment for ages 5-59, and is most widely used and most scientifically validated computerized concussion management tool, in 2013, the Journal of Athletic Training reported that up to 22-46% of healthy participants were miscategorized mostly in verbal and visual memory areas. The SCAT has a version for children, and the ACE can be used for children and adults, and in non-athlete populations. Additional tests that measure balance, such as the Balance Error Scoring System (BESS) should be included, following at least one of the above screening tools.

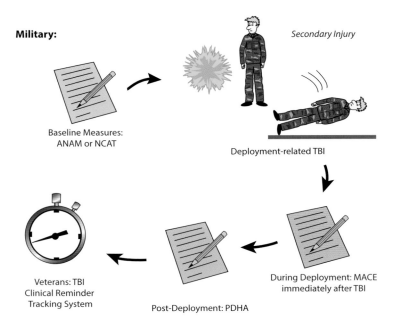

Military:

Baseline Measures:
ANAM or NCAT

Secondary Injury

Deployment-related TBI

During Deployment: MACE
immediately after TBI

Post-Deployment: PDHA

Veterans: TBI
Clinical Reminder
Tracking System

FIGURE 2.3.

There are two baseline neuropsychological tests available for the military: The Automated Neuropsychological Metric (ANAM) (Rice et al., 2011) which is required before deployment, and the Neurocognitive Assessment Tool (NCAT) program. The Military Acute Concussion Evaluation (MACE) is a screening tool for assessing concussion in a deployment setting (French et al., 2008). It takes approximately 10 minutes and should be administered by a skilled medic/corpsman or provider. Since concussion isn't always recognized in combat settings, screening of active-duty service members also occurs through post-deployment health assessments (PDHA). Positive responses on these questions should prompt a clinician interview to evaluate more fully for concussion. Veterans should be assessed through the TBI Clinical Reminder tracking system.

Victims of Intimate Partner Violence:

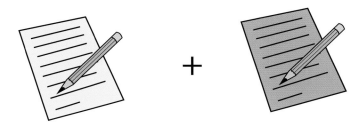

A standardized neuropsychological screening test for TBI

+

HITS
STaT
Women Abuse Screen Tool
HELPS

FIGURE 2.4.

When someone has suffered from an intimate partner violence (IPV)-related traumatic brain injury (TBI), traditional screening is not adequate. IPV-specific screening tools have been used in a number of studies with highest levels of sensitivity and specificity assigned to Hurt, Insult, Threaten, Scream (HITS) (Sherin et al., 1998), Ongoing Abuse Screen/Ongoing Violence Assessment Tool (Weiss et al., 2003), Slapped, Threatened, and Throw (STaT) (Paranjape et al., 2006), Humiliation, Afraid, Rape, Kick (Sohal et al., 2007), and Women Abuse Screen Tool (MacMillan et al., 2009). HELPS has also been indicated for IPV-related TBI (Picard et al., 1991). (H=hit in the head, E=emergency room treatment, L=loss of consciousness, P=problems with concentration and memory, S=sickness/physical problems following injury). When IPV-related TBI is suspected, an IPV-specific screening evaluation in addition to traditional standardized neurospsychological screening for TBI is recommended.

NEUROIMAGING FOR THE DETECTION OF TRAUMATIC BRAIN INJURY

Neuroimaging Modality	Measures	Results	Effectiveness	Challenges/ Future Directions
Computed Tomography (CT)	Skull fracture, intracranial hemorrhage, and brain edema	Established imaging modality for acute clinical setting	Rules out severe complications	Only about 10% of scans reveal abnormalities from mTBIs
Magnetic Resonance Imaging (MRI)	Skull fracture, intracranial hemorrhage, and brain edema	Established imaging modality for acute clinical setting	Rules out severe complications	Only about 30% of scans reveal abnormalities from mTBIs
High-Resolution Magnetic Resonance Imaging (MRI)	Effects of mTBI on cortical thickness	Widespread cortical thinning in frontal, parietal, temporal and occipital lobes in children 3 years post-TBI	May be useful tool in the assessment of more chronic stages following mTBI	Future research is needed to detect more acute structural brain changes following mTBI
Susceptibility-weighted Imaging (SWI)	Grandient-recalled echo MRI pulse sequence measures susceptibility differences between tissues	Identifies microhemorrhages resulting from mTBI microhemorrhages resulting	Possible to detect more subtle-intensity changes in sensitized images than conventional analysis techniques	Not as effective as Diffusion Tensor Imaging
Functional Magnetic Resonance Imaging (fMRI) and resting state fMRI (rsfMRI)	Cerebral blood flow using the blood oxygen level-dependent contrast that results from the paramagnetic deoxyhemoglobin in blood	Altered activation patterns have been observed in patients with mTBI and repetitive TBI	Severity of post-concussive symptoms is associated with atypical higher activation patterns in fMRI and patients with mTBI have shown disruption of the default mode network (DMN) in rsfMRI	Research in this area is expected to grow over the next few years. The effectiveness of these techniques for diagnosis, prognosis, and treatment monitoring is promising.
Dynamic Susceptibility Contrast MRI (DSC-MRI)	Dynamically quantifies cerebral hemodynamics and regional cerebral blood flow (rCBF)	In patients with mTBI, decreased brain perfusion was found in several brain regions compared to controls	DCE-MRI has the potential to detect breaks in the blood–brain barrier (BBB) accurately	Further cross-sectional and longitudinal studies on mTBI are needed to estimate the role of DCE-MRI in the diagnosis and prognosis of mTBI

FIGURE 2.5.

NEUROIMAGING FOR THE DETECTION OF TRAUMATIC BRAIN INJURY

Neuroimaging Modality	Measures	Results	Effectiveness	Challenges/ Future Directions
Arterial Spin Labeling (ASL)	Noninvasive variant of MR perfusion imaging that uses water in the blood as an internal contrast agent	Patients with a history of mTBI had reduced perfusion in the thalamus and posterior cingulate cortices	Noninvasive method for studying patients in the chronic stage of TBI	Technical improvements suggest that it is a promising tool for the evaluation of patients with mTBI
Diffusion Tensor Imaging (DTI)	Diffusion properties of water molecules in the brain	Repetitive TBIs can have accumulative effects on neural structures measured by DTI	Since 2002, DTI measures have been found to correlate with postconcussive symptoms and cognitive performance	Novel DTI sequences such as high angular resolution diffusion imaging (HARDI) and novel analysis tools are currently being developed
MR Spectroscopy (MRS)	The concentration of metabolites in human tissue based on the resonance frequency of certain isotopes	Adult patients with history of mTBI have a decrease in N-acetyl aspartame in several brain regions	Applied to TBI, MRS has shown significant changes in brain metabolism in the acute phase	Future studies will have to define standardized protocols for MRS analyses, as there are many ways to measure metabolite concentrations
Positron-emission tomography (PET)	Uses markers labeled with radioactive isotopes to detect increase in binding or uptake of the marker	FDG-PET studies consistently report hypometabolism in frontal and temporal regions	FDG-PET is effective in studying mTBI, and Tau ligands are effective in studying CTE	High costs and the exposure to ionizing radiation
Single-photon emission computer tomography (SPECT)	Used the distribution of an injected radionuclide to quantify regional cerebral blood flow (rCBF)	Hypoperfusion of several brain regions in retired NFL players	MRI and neuropsychological tests fail to correlate well with SPECT	In a clinical setting the use of SPECT alone is not believed to be sufficient in the evaluation of a patient with mTBI, because of a lack of sensitivity

Chapter 2: Screening for the Occurrence, Severity, Symptoms, and Environmental Risk Factors
Associated with Traumatic Brain Injury

37

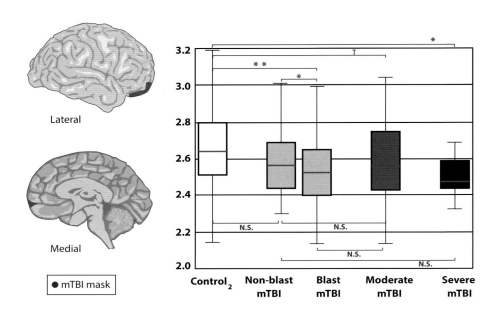

Lateral

Medial

● mTBI mask

Control₂ Non-blast mTBI Blast mTBI Moderate mTBI Severe mTBI

FIGURE 2.6.

In a recent study, magnetic resonance imaging (MRI) was used to distinguish differences in cortical thickness in US military service members who experienced blast-induced mTBIs versus non-blast induced TBIs of various severities. Participants had chronic TBI symptoms for at least 3 months post-injury. Blast-induced mTBIs resulted in significantly thinner regions in the frontal pole, rostral middle frontal cortex, pars orbitalis, lateral and medial orbitofrontal cortex, and superior frontal cortex (Eierud et al., Society for Neuroscience Abstract, 2016). There was no significant difference between mild and moderate TBI. No difference was detected in cortical thickness between severe TBI and any other TBI cohort. Cortical thinning in the right orbitofrontal cortex was observed in all TBI groups, including mTBI compared to the control group. The study results, while preliminary, suggest that MRI may be sensitive to the detection of blast-induced mTBIs.

MINOR/MILD TBI   **MODERATE TBI**   **SEVERE TBI**

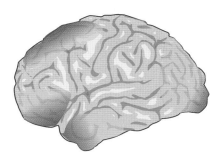
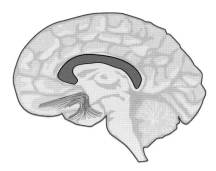

Lateral   Medial

FIGURE 2.7.

Conventional neuroimaging has low sensitivity to identify pathological changes in less severe traumatic brain injury (TBI). Diffusion tensor imaging (DTI) is a neuroimaging technique for studying in vivo the anatomy and integrity of white matter tracts in the human brain, and may provide more sensitive measurements of discrete axonal injury in TBI compared to other methods, in both the acute and chronic phase, following injury. DTI is particularly sensitive to changes in the microstructure of frontal white matter, providing a valuable biomarker of the severity of TBI and a prognostic indicator of recovery of function. DTI can be used to map white matter lesions onto individual tracts (Zapalla et al., 2012). DTI tractography has shown axonal shearing of the corpus callosum (Lee et al., 2005). There is a significant correlation between fractional anisotropy (FA) measurement of this tract and post-concussion symptoms, such as poor memory/concentration and headache/dizziness (Wilde et al., 2008). DTI has been an important imaging tool to study mTBI because it is the main imaging tool to reveal diffuse axonal injury, the main injury observed in mTBI. Future directions for research include increasing the sensitivity and specificity of DTI findings in mTBI. Here, there are three important foci: (1) technical improvements in DTI, (2) novel diffusion measures, and (3) innovative analysis techniques that reflect a move toward more individualized medicine.

Screening MRI for Intracranial Hemorrhage

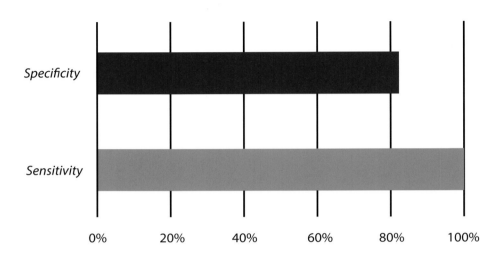

FIGURE 2.8.

Computerized tomography (CT) has been the gold standard for assessing infants with potential abusive head trauma (AHT) because the scan can be completed quickly and does not require sedation; however, there is increasing concern about the radiation exposure linked to cancer, particularly in young children. Conventional magnetic resonance imaging (MRI) is challenging for this population due to the need for sedation, which elicits concerns about the effects of anesthesia on the developing brain. In contrast, rapid-sequence MRI is a fast T2-weighted sequence that eliminates the costs and risks associated with sedation of infants, along with concerns about radiation exposure. In a recent study by Flom et al., a novel screening MRI protocol was designed and tested to determine if it could identify intracranial hemorrhage in well-appearing infants at risk for AHT, thus reducing the need for exposure to CT. For the validation cohort, the sensitivity of the screening MRI for intracranial hemorrhage was 100%, while specificity was 83%. The novel MRI technique is suggested as an appropriate screening tool for well-appearing infants, so that brain injury is not missed, and AHT is not misdiagnosed.

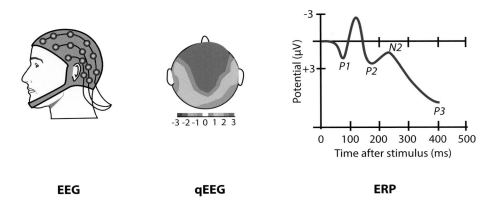

EEG   **qEEG**   **ERP**

FIGURE 2.9.

The electroencephalogram (EEG), and related neuroimaging techniques have been used to detect sport-related traumatic brain injuries on the sidelines. While EEG provides a reading of electrical activity on the scalp that originates from within neurons, Quantitative EEG (qEEG) has effectively been used to detect changes in brain electrical processing following a TBI, by recording EEG activity from large arrays of electrodes on the scalp (Gosselin et al., 2009). Importantly, qEEG measures continue to demonstrate differences in brain signals up to a week later, for sports-related TBIs compared to controls, even when behavioral differences are not present (McCrea et al., 2010). Similar results have been reported for up to 45 days post injury (Barr et al., 2012). qEEG was much more effective in predicting when concussed athletes were ready to return to play with up to 80% accuracy for mild and moderate TBIs (Prichep et al., 2013). Event related potential (ERP) has also been successful in identifying relationships between brain-behavior measures in concussed versus nonconcussed athletes (Broglio et al., 2011).

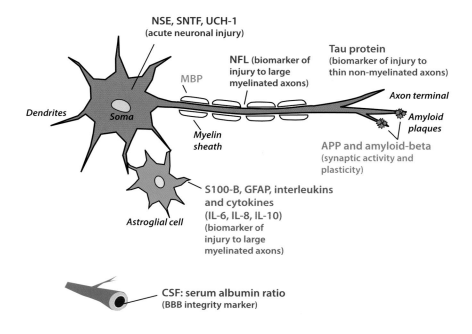

FIGURE 2.10.

There are several biomarkers in cerebral spinal fluid (CSF), blood, and saliva that can be used to detect the occurrence of, and monitor the severity of traumatic brain injury in living patients. The biomarkers are typically used to track injuries in 6 main areas indicative of traumatic brain injury: 1) Blood Brain Barrier (BBB) integrity (increase in the CSF: serum albumin ratio suggests BBB damage), 2) Acute neuronal injury, 3) Astroglial injury, 4) Axonal injury (injury to large myelinated axons and injury to thin nonmyelinated axons), 5) Neuroinflammation, and 6) Damage to synaptic activity/plasticity (Zetterberg et al., 2013). NSE =γ-enolase, SNTF = calpain-cleaved αll-spectrin N-terminal fragment, UCH-1 = ubiquitin carboxyl-terminal hydrolase isoenzyme L1, MBP = myelin basic protein, NFL = neurofilament light polypeptide, GFAP = glial fibrillary acidic protein, APP = amyloid precursor protein, S100B = S100 calcium-binding protein B, IL-6 = interleukin-6, IL-8 = interleukin-8, IL-10 = interleukin-10.

BIOMARKERS FOR THE DETECTION OF MTBI AND CTE

Biomarker Assessment	Associated With TBI Severity	Associated With Cognitive Symptoms	Detect mTBI	Found in CSF / Blood?
Albumin	Yes	N/A	No	Both - ratio
Cytokines	Yes	Yes (animals)	N/A	Both
NFL	Yes (corresponds to # of hits in boxers)	N/A	Yes, most sensitive to axonal injury	Both
NSE	Yes and mortality	Yes	Yes	Both
S100B	Yes (correlated with abnormal CT/MRI findings)	Yes	No, GFAP is better	Both
Tau	Yes	Yes	Yes	Both
GFAP	Yes	Yes	Yes, peaks 20 hours post-injury	Both
UCH-L1	Yes	Yes	Yes, peaks 8 hours post-injury	Both
SNTF	Yes	Yes	Yes	Both

FIGURE 2.11.

Biomarkers may be used to detect the occurrence of mTBI, when other methods are not ideal, such as certain types of neuroimaging. Plasma levels of calpain-cleaved αll-spectrin N-terminal fragment (SNTF) were measured in CT-negative mTBI patients who underwent diffusion tensor imaging (DTI) and cognitive testing. SNTF was significantly elevated in patients with mTBI. Levels of SNTF were associated with differences in fiber density, axonal diameter, and myelination obtained from diffusion tensor imaging (DTI) in several brain regions. Glial fibrillary acidic protein (GFAP) can be measured to assess neurological damage, if the sample is taken early after injury. If too much time has passed, ubiquitin carboxyl-terminal hydrolase isoenzyme L1 (UCH-L1) is a better assessment of neurological damage. For chronic traumatic encephalopathy (CTE), two CSF biomarkers that have been the focus of research are the axonal proteins: tau and NFL (neurofilament light polypeptide). In a longitudinal study in amateur boxers, marked increases in CSF NFL and tau were observed after sparring bouts. In 78 former NFL players, significantly higher levels of plasma exosomal tau was detected compared to 16 controls ($p<0.0001$). Within the former NFL athlete group, higher exosomal tau was associated with significantly worse performance on memory tests and psychomotor speed (Zetterberg et al., 2013).

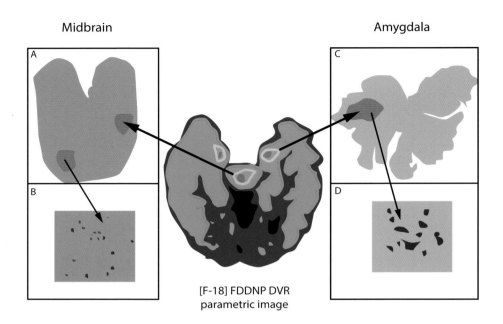

Midbrain   Amygdala

[F-18] FDDNP DVR
parametric image

FIGURE 2.12.

While there is no definitive clinical diagnosis of CTE at the present time, these tau-sensitive brain imaging agents may be able to detect the disease in living people. Early detection would allow for more effective management and treatment strategies. Positron-emission tomography (PET) can be used in conjunction with tau tracers to detect tau pathology in individuals suspected of having Chronic Traumatic Encephalopathy (CTE), such as 2-I1{6-[(2-[F-18] flouroethyl)(methyl)amino]-2-naphthyl}ethylidene)malononitrile, or [F-18]FDDNP. In a recent study, FDDNP was used to assess tau pathology in a small group of football players suspected of having CTE. [F-18] FDDNP signals were higher in all subcortical areas known to produce tau deposits, compared to healthy controls (Barrio et al., 2015). In a follow-up study, imaging patterns of [F-18] FDDNP were significantly different in retired NFL players suspected of having CTE, compared to those with Alzheimer's Disease (AD) or normal aging (Barrio et al., 2015). A-D show results of tau immunohistochemistry and demonstrate that in the mTBI group, areas of increased [F-18] FDDNP signal in the amygdala and dorsal midbrain (middle image) coincide with presence of tau deposits in the periaqueductal gray (PAG) in the dorsal midbrain (A and B) and in amygdala (C and D) paired helical filament (PHF)-tau distribution observed at autopsy in subjects with a confirmed diagnosis of CTE (Barrio et al., 2015).

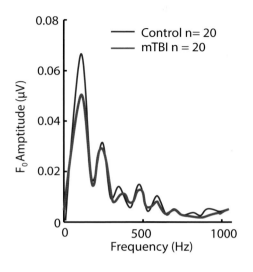

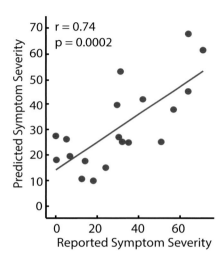

FIGURE 2.13.

Traumatic brain injury, even when mild, can result in compromised sound processing. In a recent study (Kraus et al., 2016), researchers examined whether sports-related concussion in children (mean age 13.5 years old) results in disruption of the neural processing of the fundamental frequency, a key component for understanding speech. Children who have sustained a concussion exhibit a signature neural profile, resulting in an impaired representation of the fundamental frequency, and smaller, slower neural responses. Concussed children (shown in red) have smaller responses to the pitch of a talker's voice than their non-concussed peers (shown in black). In the study, neural processing of sound correctly identified 90% of concussion cases and cleared 95% of control cases. Partial recovery of auditory processing was observed as concussion symptoms declined, suggesting that this approach may serve as a scalable biological marker for sports-related concussions, at least in children. Further testing is needed to examine whether findings extend to other age groups and non-athlete related concussions.

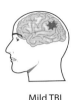

Mild TBI

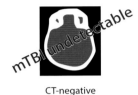

CT-negative

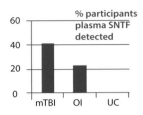

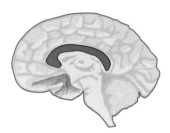

Abnormalities detected with DTI

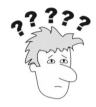

Cognitive impairment
3 months post injury

FIGURE 2.14.

In a recent study, plasma levels of calpain-cleaved αll-spectrin N-terminal fragment (SNTF) were measured in athletes with mTBI, athletes with orthopedic injury (OI), or healthy controls who underwent diffusion tensor imaging (DTI) and cognitive testing (Siman et al., 2013). All patients with mTBI were CT-negative after injury. Levels of SNTF were significantly higher in patients with mTBI compared to participants with OI, or controls. Increased levels of SNTF correlated with differences in fiber density, axonal diameter, and myelination obtained from diffusion tensor imaging (DTI) in the uncinate fasciculus and corpus callosum. Increased levels of SNTF were also associated with cognitive impairment 3 months later.

BIOMARKERS FOR MONITORING RECOVERY TIME FOR TRAUMATIC BRAIN INJURY

Blood tau measured
6, 24, and 72 hours
post-concussion

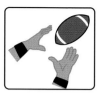

Ready to return to play

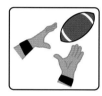

Return to play in more
than 10 days

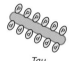

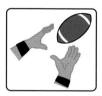

Return to play in 10 days
or less

FIGURE 2.15.

Despite millions of sports-related concussions that occur annually in the US, there is no reliable blood-based test to predict recovery, or athlete readiness to return to play. In a recent study, researchers at the National Institute of Health (NIH) discovered that the blood protein tau may be a potential objective tool to assess athlete recovery and the most appropriate time to return to play (Bendlin and Makdissi, 2017). A group of 632 athletes in high-contact sports (soccer, football, basketball, hockey, and lacrosse) from the University of Rochester underwent blood plasma sampling and cognitive testing to establish a baseline. After being followed throughout the season, 43 athletes were diagnosed with concussion. A control group of 37 teammate athletes without concussion, and a group of 21 healthy non-athletes were included in the study. Following a sports-related concussion, blood was sampled from both concussed and control athletes at six hours, 24 hours, 72 hours, and seven days post-concussion. Concussed athletes who needed a longer recovery time before returning to play (more than ten days post-concussion) had higher tau concentrations overall at six, 24, and 72-hours post-concussion compared to athletes who were able to return to play in 10 days or less. Observed alterations in tau levels occurred in both male and female athletes, and across the various sports studied. The findings suggest that changes in tau measured as early as six hours post-concussion may provide important clinical information about recovery times and safe return to play.

Chapter 2: Screening for the Occurrence, Severity, Symptoms, and Environmental Risk Factors
Associated with Traumatic Brain Injury

47

Risk Factors for TBI

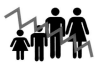
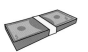
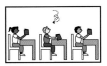

Dysfunctional Family   Economic Factors   ADHD

Risk Factors for SIS

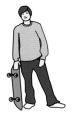

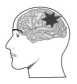

First concussion   American football   Male gender   Young age (16-19 yrs)

FIGURE 2.16.

Some of the most common risk factors for traumatic brain injury in adolescents are: low socioeconomic status, a dysfunctional family environment, and the diagnosis of Attention Deficit Hyperactivity Disorder (ADHD) (Chasle et al., 2016). In a recent study, 675 adolescents/children with mTBI compared to controls were observed for ADHD. In the mTBI cohort, 18% were diagnosed with ADHD compared to 11% in controls (Chasle et al., 2016). The results suggest that pre-existing psychiatric conditions such as ADHD, and other environmental stressors, may contribute to the prevalence of TBI in adolescents. The greatest risk factor associated with Second Impact Syndrome (SIS) is premature return to sports activity after suffering an initial traumatic brain injury (TBI), no matter how mild (McLendon et al., 2016). While the literature on SIS is scarce, other risk factors associated with this devastating condition are: American football, male gender, and young age (Bey and Ostick, 2008).

Percentage of Prior Opportunities Associated with Abusive Head Trauma in Children

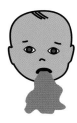

Vomiting
31.6%

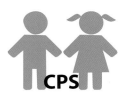

Prior CPS contact
20%

Bruising
11.7%

FIGURE 2.17.

Infants with minor abusive injuries are at risk for more serious abusive injury, including Abusive Head Trauma (AHT). In a recent study of 232 infants diagnosed with AHT, 10% died, while 32% had a total of 120 prior opportunities to detect AHT (Letson et al., 2016). Prior opportunity was defined as prior evaluation by a medical or child protective services(CPS) professional when the symptoms and/or referral could be consistent with abuse, but the diagnosis was not made, or an alternative explanation was given. The most common prior opportunities involved vomiting (31.6%), prior CPS contact (20%), and bruising (11.7%) (Letson et al., 2016). Improvements in earlier detection of AHT, and the early signs associated with it, may prevent additional injuries and infant death.

CHAPTER 3

Differential Diagnosis: Neuropsychiatric Conditions Associated with Traumatic Brain Injury

In Chapter 3, we begin by highlighting potential neurobiological regions of damage caused by traumatic brain injury (TBI) that are associated with comorbid neuropsychiatric conditions such as pseudobulbar affect, depression, anxiety, mania, post traumatic stress disorder (PTSD), personality disorders, psychosis, and aggression. We also address neurological consequences associated with TBI, such as sleep disturbances, and cognitive impairment.

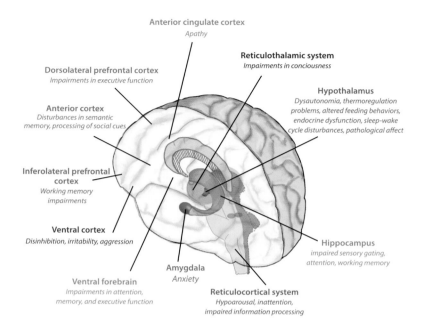

FIGURE 3.1.

Traumatic Brain Injury (TBI) is associated with multiple neuropsychiatric sequelae, including problems with cognition, emotion, and behavior. Although TBI can affect any area of the brain, there is a relatively consistent pattern of regional cerebral vulnerability to injury, whether mild or more severe. That pattern of regional vulnerability underlies the types of neuropsychiatric problems commonly experienced by patients with TBI (Silver et al., 2009). Eleven brain regions are depicted in the figure above, with the most common neuropsychiatric symptoms associated with damage to each. Neuropsychiatric symptoms of patients with TBI may not fit neatly into DSM diagnostic criteria, however, 44% of individuals with TBI-related psychiatric diagnoses have 2 or more disorders. Three-fourths of veterans diagnosed with TBI are also diagnosed with PTSD, and one-half are also diagnosed with depression. Patients with major depression following TBI are 8X more likely to have comorbid anxiety compared to patients with TBI and no depression (Silver et al., 2009).

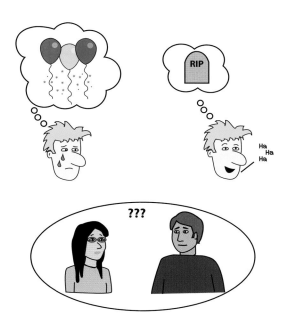

FIGURE 3.2.

Pseudobulbar affect (PBA) is an emotional expression disorder, characterized by uncontrolled crying or laughing which may be disproportionate or inappropriate to the social context. PBA can accompany a variety of neurodegenerative diseases and neurological injuries, such as Traumatic Brain Injury (TBI). Terminology for PBA has been varied and confusing, such as: involuntary emotional expression disorder (IEED), emotional lability, emotional dysregulation, pathological laughter and crying (PLC), emotional dysregulation, emotional incontinence, and emotionalism. The inconsistent use of terminology has led to debate and confusion in the field. Guidelines have been suggested by Cummings et al. (2006) to provide diagnostic criteria for this disorder, and to use a medically accurate and unifying term to encompass disorders of emotional affect—such as IEED.

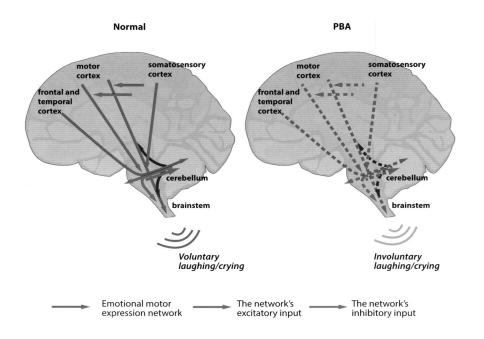

FIGURE 3.3.

The underlying mechanism in PBA appears to be lack of voluntary control, also termed disinhibition; however, the pathways are complex and not yet completely understood. Detailed reviews of the widespread anatomical and neurophysiological abnormalities found by neuroimaging and neurophysiological studies in patients with PBA suggest that the cerebellum appears to play a much greater role in PBA than was hypothesized a few years ago (Parvizi et al., 2006; Miller et al., 2011). One hypothesis is that the cerebellum plays a key role in modulating emotional responses so as to keep them appropriate to the social situation and to the patient's mood based on input from the cerebral cortex. Disruption of the corticopontine-cerebellar circuits results in impairment of this cerebellar modulation, causing PBA (Parvizi et al., 2009; Miller et al., 2011). The primary neurotransmitters believed to be involved in PBA are serotonin and glutamate. The role of serotonin in corticolimbic or cerebellar pathways most likely contributes to its impact on PBA, whereas modulation of glutamate may have widespread effects (Miller et al., 2011).

DIAGNOSIS OF PSEUDOBULBAR AFFECT (PBA) IN PATIENTS WITH TRAUMATIC BRAIN INJURY

Table 2 Diagnostic criteria for pseudobulbar affect
Poeck
The emotional response is situationally inappropriate
The patient's feelings and the affective response are not closely related
The duration and severity of the episodes cannot be controlled by the patient
Expression of the emotion does not lead to a feeling of relief
Cummings: Necessary elements of the episodes
A change from previous emotional responses
Inconsistent with or disproportionate to mood
Not dependent on a stimulus, or excessive relative to that stimulus
Cause significant distress or social/occupational impairment
Not accounted for by another psychiatric or neurologic disorder
Not due to a drug

FIGURE 3.4.

Pseudobulbar affect (PBA) disorder has often been judged by a clinician in an informal manner, as part of a neurological evaluation, and it is most commonly misidentified as a mood disorder, particularly depression or bipolar disorder (Ahmed et al., 2013). PBA may be more objectively measured by published scales, such as The Center for Neurologic Study- Lability Scale (CNS-LS), or the Pathological Laughter and Crying Scale (PLACS). The PLACS has shown excellent interrater and test-retest reliability. Both scales have been used in studies of treatment of PBA. The most current diagnostic criteria for PBA, according to Poeck (1969), and Cummings et al. (2006), are listed in the table.

DEPRESSION IN PATIENTS WITH TRAUMATIC BRAIN INJURY

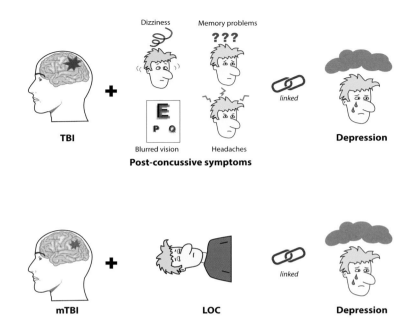

FIGURE 3.5.

Depression is the most common psychiatric complication of TBI. Patients with TBI remain at elevated risk of depression for decades post-injury and 90% of patients with TBI and major depressive disorder (MDD) experienced the onset of depression post-TBI. Patients with mild traumatic brain injury (mTBI) and depression are more likely to report loss of consciousness (LOC) at the time of injury. Depression following TBI is associated with more severe post-concussive symptoms, including headache, blurred vision, dizziness, and memory impairment (Silver et al., 2009).

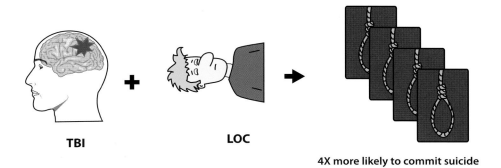

TBI

LOC

4X more likely to commit suicide

FIGURE 3.6.

Suicide rates among patients with TBI are higher than in the general population. Patients with TBI and loss of consciousness have 4X greater likelihood of attempting suicide than the general population. 10–33% of patients report suicidal ideation 1 year post-TBI. 15% of patients attempt suicide by 5 years post-TBI. Women who have experienced IPV have significantly higher rates of suicide than women who have not experienced an abusive relationship (Golding, 1999). Data on suicide from intimate partner violence (IPV)-related TBI specifically, is lacking.

MANIA IN PATIENTS WITH TRAUMATIC BRAIN INJURY

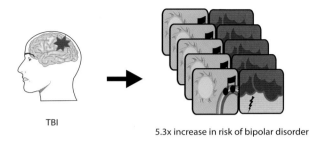

TBI

5.3x increase in risk of bipolar disorder

Mania symptoms following TBI

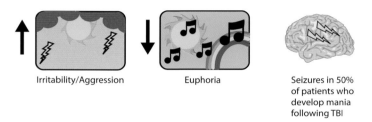

Irritability/Aggression

Euphoria

Seizures in 50% of patients who develop mania following TBI

FIGURE 3.7.

Following traumatic brain injury (TBI), the risk of bipolar disorder increases 5.3-fold (Rogers et al., 2009); however, it is sometimes difficult to differentiate whether mania symptoms are specifically related to the TBI. Mania due to TBI should be suspected if the symptoms are in close temporal relationship and in the absence of other etiology. Other indicators of TBI-related mania are atypical age of onset of symptoms and/or lack of family history. TBI-related mania symptoms typically present more as aggressive and irritable moods, with less euphoria. Seizures develop in 50% of patients who develop mania following TBI. There is some evidence for manic symptoms following limbic-connected right hemisphere lesions (Starkstein et al., 1987), and temporal basal polar lesions (Pope et al., 1998).

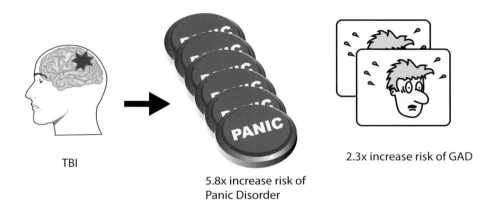

TBI

5.8x increase risk of
Panic Disorder

2.3x increase risk of GAD

FIGURE 3.8.

TBI increases the risk of Generalized Anxiety Disorder (GAD) by 2.3X, and panic disorder by 5.8X (van Reekum et al., 2000). Fifteen years after TBI, 44% of patients met diagnostic criteria for GAD, suggesting that TBI patients remain at an elevated risk for GAD for years following injury (Hoofien et al., 2001). GAD co-morbidity was negatively associated with patient recovery (Hoofien et al., 2001). In most cases, panic disorder manifests over 10 years following TBI, suggesting that the disorder is a slowly evolving reaction to injury (Silver et al., 2001). Anxiety in the acute stage is a significant predictor of post-concussive syndrome (PCS).

POSTTRAUMATIC STRESS DISORDER IN PATIENTS WITH TRAUMATIC BRAIN INJURY

PTSD

- Reexperiencing symptoms
- Shame
- Guilt

- Depression/anxiety
- Insomnia
- Irritability/anger
- Trouble concentrating
- Fatigue
- Hyperarousal
- Avoidance

PPCS

- Headache
- Sensitivity to light (and sound)
- Memory deficit
- Dizziness

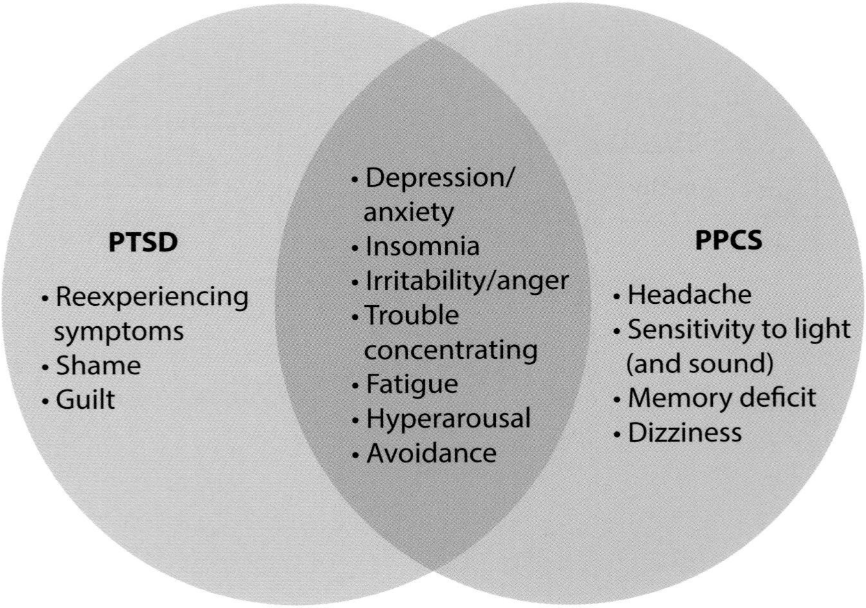

FIGURE 3.9.

Patients with traumatic brain injury (TBI) have a 5.8X increased risk for development of PTSD (van Reekum et al., 2000), and 16.5% of patients with TBI meet diagnostic criteria for PTSD (Rogers et al., 2007). Of 2,234 Operation Enduring Freedom/Operation Iraqi Freedom (OEF/OIF) veterans, 12% were diagnosed with mTBI and 11% were diagnosed with PTSD (Sayer et al., 2012; Brenner et al., 2011). For victims of intimate partner violence (IPV), women with TBI reported to have greater levels of PTSD symptomology than women without TBI. In a study of 205 women who experienced IPV-related TBI, 56% had PTSD. Conversely, the combat or abusive environment may independently increase the risk for both TBI and PTSD. Unfortunately, common brain areas are implicated in both PTSD and post-concussive syndrome (McAllister et al., 2011), raising challenges when it comes to differential diagnosis.

PERSONALITY CHANGES/DISORDERS IN PATIENTS WITH TRAUMATIC BRAIN INJURY

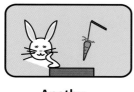

Apathy

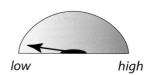

low   *high*

Emotional Stability

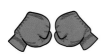

Reduced anger control/increased aggression

Impulsivity

Impaired social judgment

FIGURE 3.10.

Approximately one-third of patients with traumatic brain injury (TBI) are affected by personality changes (Diaz et al., 2012). While personality alterations can be a primary source of concern for family members, patients may not recognize these changes (McAllister et al., 2011). Personality changes can persist for years post-injury and can include: apathy (damage to reward circuitry), emotional lability (damage to frontal cortex/limbic connections), impaired judgment (damage to prefrontal cortex), increased impulsivity (damage to frontal cortex), and irritability (damage to orbitofrontal cortex) (McAllister et al., 2011).

AGGRESSION IN PATIENTS WITH TRAUMATIC BRAIN INJURY

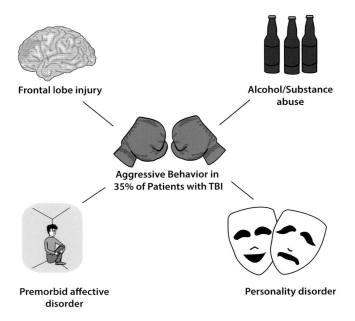

Frontal lobe injury

Alcohol/Substance abuse

Aggressive Behavior in 35% of Patients with TBI

Premorbid affective disorder

Personality disorder

FIGURE 3.11.

Aggression is a commonly reported behavioral symptom of traumatic brain injury (TBI), most typically associated with moderate and severe injuries. In one study, 34% of patients with TBI exhibited aggressive behavior within six months (Tateno et al., 2011). Hostility, temper outbursts, and poor self-control may be present for decades following TBI. Risk factors for aggression following TBI involve: frontal lobe injury, premorbid affective disorder, personality disorder, and alcohol or substance abuse (Riggio, 2010). Presence of agitation during acute recovery predicts poorer psychological adjustment and long-term outcomes (Vaishnavi et al., 2009). Damage to the limbic system, orbitofrontal cortex, left anteromedial frontal lobe, and anterior cingulate gyri has been particularly associated with aggressive behavior (Grafman et al., 1996).

THE TBI-VIOLENCE CYCLE

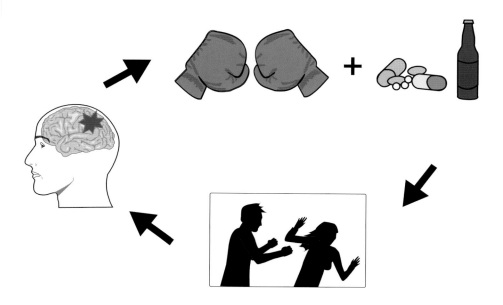

FIGURE 3.12.

The aggression and violence associated with traumatic brain injury (TBI) suggests that brain trauma may also be a risk factor for intimate partner violence (IPV). TBI is associated with an increase in physical and verbal aggression and criminal behavior. In a meta-analysis including six studies, 53.6% of 222 IPV offenders had a history of TBI, which was significantly higher than the general population (38.5%) (Farrer et al., 2012). Other factors may contribute (e.g., substance abuse). Further research is needed to elucidate the relationship between alcohol/substance abuse, TBI, and IPV.

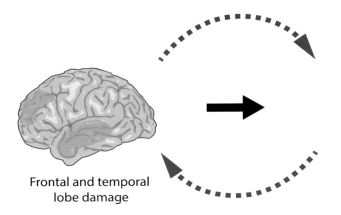

Frontal and temporal
lobe damage

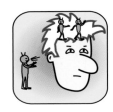

60% increase in risk
of schizophrenia

FIGURE 3.13.

TBI increases the risk of developing schizophrenia by 60% and is possibly associated with frontal and temporal lobe damage (Molloy et al., 2011). Risk is typically higher for those who have a family history of schizophrenia, suggesting a genetic-environmental interaction (Molloy et al., 2011). There is a wide range of the delay in the onset of psychotic symptoms following TBI; however, research indicates that the average onset is approximately 4 years post-injury (Achte et al., 1991; Fujii et al., 2001; Sachdev et al., 2001). Studies have reported that 33–58% of patients with TBI-related psychosis experience seizures (Fujii et al., 2001; Hillbom et al., 1960). Post-TBI schizophrenia is difficult to diagnose because patients with schizophrenia may be at a higher risk of sustaining a TBI during their lifetime. Schizophrenia-like psychosis occurs 12X more frequently in patients with seizure disorder compared to the general population (McKenna et al., 1985; Davison et al., 1983).

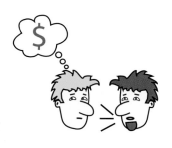
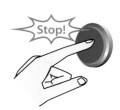
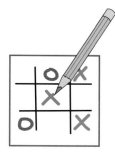
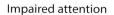

| Impaired attention | Impaired inhibition of incorrect responses | Impaired recognition of mistakes |

FIGURE 3.14.

Cognitive deficits are the most common complaint following TBI, and tend to persist for decades following injury. Deficits may include difficulties with: attention/sustained attention (Frencham et al., 2005; Peskind et al, 2011), executive function (Frencham et al., 2005; Peskind et al., 2011), working memory (Frencham et al., 2005; Peskind et al., 2011), language/communication (Levin and Chapman et al., 1998), processing speed, impaired inhibition of incorrect responses, impaired recognition of mistakes (Frencham et al., 2005; Peskind et al., 2011), verbal memory, and visual memory (Frencham et al., 2005).

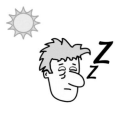

Excessive daytime
sleepiness

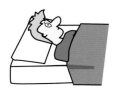

Insomnia

Impaired sleep
wake cycle

Obstructive sleep apnea

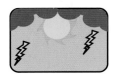

Irritability/Aggression

FIGURE 3.15.

Traumatic brain injury (TBI) is associated with sleep disturbances. Recently, systematic and prospective studies have reported TBI-associated sleep disruption. In one study, 72% of patients with TBI had a sleep–wake disorder, irrespective of the localization or severity of the trauma (Baumann, 2012). Hypersomnia was found in 22% of patients with TBI 6 months post-injury (Baumann et al., 2007). Excessive daytime sleepiness and fatigue was observed in 55% of patients with TBI (Masel et al., 2001). A prospective study based on sleep questionnaires found a high prevalence (30%) of insomnia and poor sleep quality in patients after TBI (Fichtenberg et al., 2002). In another study, 36% of patients with TBI and complaints of insomnia had circadian rhythm disorders (Ayalon et al., 2007). Obstructive sleep apnea and narcolepsy are also not uncommon (Collen et al., 2012). Insomnia in patients with TBI is associated with headaches, depressive symptoms, and irritability. Unrecognized or untreated sleep disorders may worsen outcomes and increase disability from TBI. In the military, combat-related TBI injury type (blunt injury) predicted the development of obstructive sleep apnea (Collen et al., 2012).

CHAPTER 4

Current Treatment Approaches for Neuropsychiatric Symptoms Associated with Traumatic Brain Injury

In Chapter 4, we present a checklist for treating patients with traumatic brain injury (TBI), that addresses their physical, emotional, and cognitive needs. We offer general guidelines on pharmacological treatment of neuropsychiatric conditions associated with TBI, and we present traditional methods for the treatment of these conditions (e.g., transcranial magnetic stimulation for treatment-resistant depression). We also discuss alternative/novel treatments for many neuropsychiatric conditions associated with TBI, such as headache, sleep disruptions, post-concussive symptoms, depression, and posttraumatic stress disorder (PTSD).

CHECKLIST FOR TREATING PATIENTS WITH TRAUMATIC BRAIN INJURY

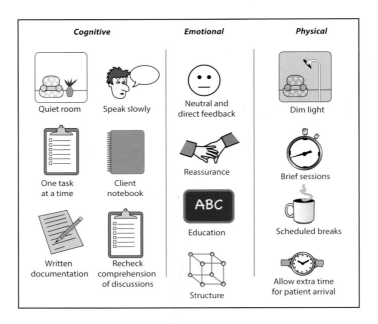

	Cognitive	Emotional	Physical
	Quiet room	Neutral and direct feedback	Dim light
	Speak slowly		
	One task at a time	Reassurance	Brief sessions
	Client notebook		
	Written documentation	Education	Scheduled breaks
	Recheck comprehension of discussions	Structure	Allow extra time for patient arrival

FIGURE 4.1.

When treating patients with traumatic brain injury (TBI), taking several actions in the cognitive, emotional, and physical realms, to make treatment sessions more comfortable for the patient is highly recommended (Murray et al., 2016). For cognitive challenges after TBI: therapy sessions should occur in a quiet room with limited distractions; speed of discussion should be slowed to allow for processing; only one task should be presented at a time; the patient should be offered extra time for responses; comprehension of discussions should be confirmed with the patient; written documentation should be provided to supplement verbal discussions and help the patient retain information; the client should be encouraged to keep a notebook for remembering; assistance should be given to help the patient organize and prioritize tasks; and finally several solutions for problem-solving should be provided. For TBI-related emotional challenges, minimize anxiety for the patient with reassurance, education, and structure. In addition, provide neutral, direct feedback for the patient. For TBI-related physical challenges, allow extra time for client, keep the environment quiet, minimize bright lights, keep client sessions brief, and schedule rest periods/breaks (Murray et al., 2016).

GENERAL GUIDELINES FOR PHARMACOLOGICAL TREATMENT OF PATIENTS WITH TRAUMATIC BRAIN INJURY

DO	DON'T
Start low	Anticholinergic agents
Titrate slow	Sedating agents
	Agents that lower seizure threshold
	Agents with a risk of Extra Pyramidal Symptoms (EPS) and Tardive Dyskinesia (TD)

FIGURE 4.2.

General guidelines are recommended for pharmacological treatment of patients with traumatic brain injury (TBI). Avoid agents with anticholinergic properties and agents that are sedating because they may worsen already impaired cognition. Avoid agents that lower the seizure threshold, because patients with TBI may already be at an increased risk for seizure activity. Animal data suggests poor neuronal recovery from conventional antipsychotics, thus they should be avoided. Patients with TBI may be more prone to Extra Pyramidal Syndrome (EPS) and tardive dyskinesia (TD), therefore agents should be avoided that are associated with a risk of EPS and TD. When prescribing any medication it is important to start low, and titrate slowly, because the injured brain may be more sensitive to psychotropic effects (Vaishnavi et al., 2009).

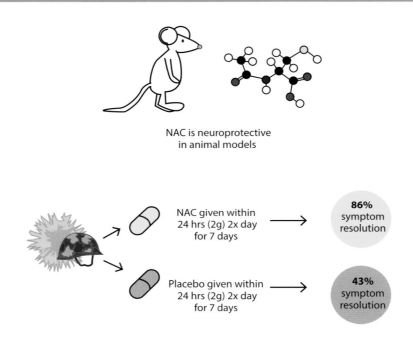

NAC is neuroprotective
in animal models

NAC given within
24 hrs (2g) 2x day
for 7 days ⟶ **86%** symptom resolution

Placebo given within
24 hrs (2g) 2x day
for 7 days ⟶ **43%** symptom resolution

FIGURE 4.3.

In a recent double-blind study, the efficacy of n-acetyl cysteine (NAC) to relieve post-concussive symptoms was examined in active duty military personnel. All participants received standard of care after experiencing a blast-induced mild traumatic brain injury (mTBI), and were randomly assigned to NAC treatment or placebo for seven days. Those in the NAC group received NAC (starting at 2g, then lowered to 1.5g) twice a day for seven days. Outcome measures consisted of: the presence of neurological and neuropsychological symptoms the day of injury and 7 days post-injury, such as dizziness, headache, hearing loss, memory loss, neurocognitive dysfunction, and sleep abnormalities. Results suggest that NAC was significantly better than placebo at resolving symptoms in active military blast-induced mTBI. NAC administration resulted in an 86% symptom resolution, compared to a 42% symptom resolution in controls (Hoffer et al., 2013).

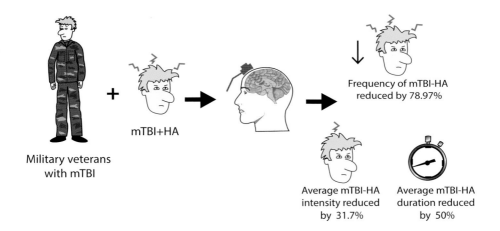

Military veterans with mTBI

mTBI+HA

Frequency of mTBI-HA reduced by 78.97%

Average mTBI-HA intensity reduced by 31.7%

Average mTBI-HA duration reduced by 50%

FIGURE 4.4.

Headache is one of the most common chronic pain conditions in patients with mild traumatic brain injury (mTBI). Conventional pharmacological treatments have not been shown to be effective at alleviating debilitating mild traumatic brain injury related headaches (MTBI-HA). Repetitive transcranial magnetic stimulation (rTMS) applies a basic electromagnetic coupling principle in which a rapid discharge of electrical current is converted into dynamic magnetic flux, allowing a localized current in the brain for neuromodulation. This technique is currently approved for treating depression in the United States, and recent meta-analysis studies have implemented rTMS in chronic pain management. In a recent small (n=6) study, 4 treatment sessions of rTMS was delivered to patients with MTBI-HA. The average headache exacerbation frequency (episodes per week) was reduced by 78.97%, with 2 patients reporting complete cessation of severe headache episodes. For those with persistent headaches, the average duration and intensity of these exacerbations was reduced by 50.0% and 31.7%, respectively (Leung et al., 2016).

PHARMACOLOGICAL AND NONPHARMACOLOGICAL TREATMENT FOR SLEEP DISTURBANCES IN PATIENTS WITH TBI

Potentially Helpful	Potentially Harmful
Sleep hygiene education	Anticholinergic agents
Melatonin supplement	Nonprescription drugs (e.g. Unisom)
Trazadone	Tricyclic antidepressants
	Benzodiazepines
	Antipsychotics

FIGURE 4.5.

For pharmacological treatment of sleep disturbances in patients with traumatic brain injury (TBI), specific guidelines should be followed, so as not to exacerbate cognitive impairment, or prevent neurological recovery. Avoid or use caution with drugs that have anticholinergic properties, nonprescription drugs (e.g., Unisom), and tricyclic antidepressants such as nortriptyline/amitriptyline. Benzodiazepines may interfere with neuroplasticity and recovery and worsen cognitive deficits. Antipsychotics may worsen obstructive sleep apnea. Potentially helpful approaches are: sleep hygiene education, melatonin supplements, and the antidepressant trazadone. Trazadone is a selective serotonin reuptake inhibitor (SSRI), that has demonstrated promising outcomes for the treatment of insomnia in patients with TBI (Larson et al., 2010). In a small study, 7 patients (6 months post-TBI) received 5 mg of melatonin for 1 month. While there were no significant improvements in sleep parameters (e.g., duration), effect sizes revealed a moderate effect on daytime alertness (Kemp et al., 2004). Melatonin has been shown to reduce latency to sleep and increase sleep efficiency in chronic and age-related insomnia (Zhdanova et al., 2001); however, more studies in patients with TBI are needed. Melatonin treatment may have additional benefits to patients with TBI. Recent studies have examined potential neuroprotective effects of melatonin treatment in animal models of TBI and have found reduced neuronal cortical apoptosis, decreased brain edema, and attenuated neurological deficits (Wu, et al., 2016).

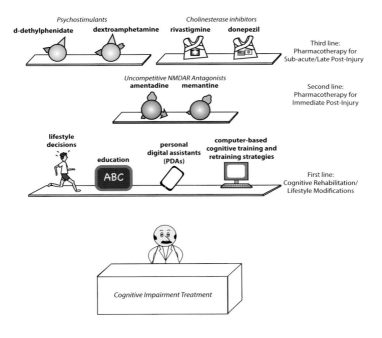

FIGURE 4.6.

The evidence base for nonpharmacologic and pharmacologic treatments has developed substantially over the last 20 years, especially in the last decade. First-line treatments for posttraumatic cognitive impairments are nonpharmacologic, including education, environmental and lifestyle modifications, and cognitive rehabilitation (Wortzel et al., 2013). Pharmacotherapies for posttraumatic cognitive impairments include uncompetitive N-methyl-d-aspartate receptor (NMDA) antagonists, medications that indirectly augment catecholaminergic or acetylcholinergic function (e.g., cholinesterase inhibitors), or agents with combinations of these properties (Wortzel et al., 2013). In addition, psychostimulants may augment cerebral catecholaminergic function, improving processing speed, arousal, attention, and memory (Vaishnavi et al., 2009). However, methylphenidate and dextroamphetamine are not recommended for patients with a history of substance abuse. In the immediate post-injury period, treatment with uncompetitive NMDA receptor antagonists reduces duration of unconsciousness, likely due to attenuation of neurotrauma-induced glutamatergic excitotoxicity from the injured brain (Wortzel et al., 2013). During the sub-acute or late post-injury periods, medications that augment cerebral acetylcholinergic functions may improve declarative memory, attention, processing speed, and executive function (Wortzel et al., 2013).

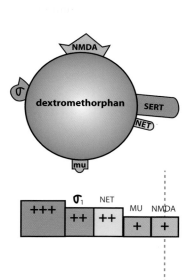

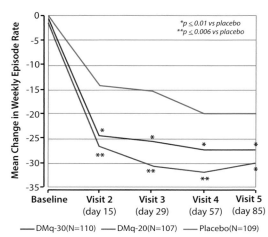

FIGURE 4.7.

Treatment of pseudobulbar affect (PBA) has primarily involved use of medications that modulate serotonergic or glutamatergic neurotransmission. Selective serotonin reuptake inhibitors, serotonin/norepinephrine reuptake inhibitors (SNRIs) and tricyclic antidepressants are used off-label to treat PBA, and have demonstrated efficacy from case studies (Kim et al., 2005), open-label trials (Seliger et al., 1992), and placebo-controlled studies (Robinson et al., 1993). Dextromethorphan/quinidine has antiglutamatergic properties and is an emerging treatment for PBA (Brooks et al., 2004; Panitch et al, 2006). Because of the rapid metabolism of dextromethorphan via CYP2D6 enzymes in the liver, it has been combined with a low dose of quinidine (a CYP2D6 inhibitor) in order to increase dextromethorphan plasma concentrations (Pope et al., 2004). While dextromethorphan might exert effects on serotonergic neurotransmission through binding at 5-HT transporters and receptors (Werling et al., 2007), its effects on glutamatergic transmission via µ-1 agonism could be particularly important for PBA treatment. Dextromethorphan binding is most prominent in the brainstem and cerebellum, key sites involved in the pathophysiology of PBA (Anderson et al., 1994) that are rich with µ receptors (Maurice et al., 2001). While the exact mechansims of dextromethorphan/quinidine in ameliorating PBA are not known, modulation of excessive glutamatergic transmission within cortico-pontine-cerebellar circuits may contribute to its benefits.

TRADITIONAL TREATMENT OF DEPRESSION IN PATIENTS WITH TBI: PHARMACOLOGICAL

Medication	Efficacy	Side Effects	Warnings
SSRIs	• First line of defense • Among SSRIs sertaline has most DA effects		• Paroxetine may impair cognition due to antimuscarinic properties
TCAs	• Less efficacy than SSRIs	• Higher risk of side effects, especially seizures / cognitive deficits	
Bupropion	• Not recommended		• Lowers seizure threshold
MAOIs	• Not recommended due to lack of efficacy data		• Dietary restrictions may be harder to follow in TBI patients
Methylphenidate	• Similar efficacy to sertaline • Improvement in cognitive deficits		

FIGURE 4.8.

Special considerations for antidepressants as treatment in patients with traumatic brain injury (TBI) are recommended. Most patients with post-TBI depression do not respond to standard antidepressant therapy. Depression resulting from a basal ganglia lesion could potentially worsen with antidepressants. Bupropion and TCAs have an increased risk of seizure associated with them. Some antidepressants may also interfere with motor function, which may already be compromised in patients with TBI. Finally, antidepressants with anticholinergic properties (e.g., paroxetine) may further impair cognition (Vaishnavi et al., 2009).

TMS treatment device

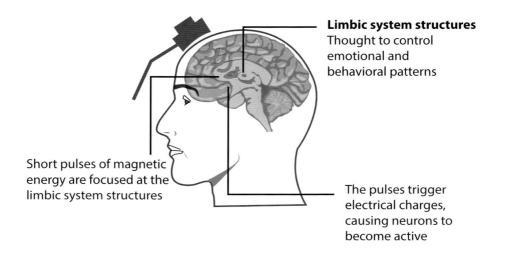

Limbic system structures
Thought to control emotional and behavioral patterns

Short pulses of magnetic energy are focused at the limbic system structures

The pulses trigger electrical charges, causing neurons to become active

FIGURE 4.9.

Up to one third of patients with traumatic brain injury (TBI) are resistant to conventional pharmacological treatment for depression. Numerous repetitive transcranial magnetic stimulation (rTMS) studies have been performed on patients with major depressive disorder (MDD) and have demonstrated positive results, suggesting that either 1) low-frequency stimulation (1 Hz) of the right dorsolateral prefrontal cortex, or 2) high frequency over the left dorsolateral prefrontal cortex, both have antidepressant effects (Brasil-Neto et al., 2003). Double-blind studies have been developed using anodal transcranial direct current stimulation (tDCS) on the left dorsolateral prefrontal cortex, with low intensities between 1 and 2mA, over 10 days or more, and have shown positive results in reducing depressive symptoms (Iannone et al., 2016). In a recent study, treatment-resistant patients who experienced repetitive head trauma underwent 20 daily sessions of bilateral rTMS treatment (4000 left-sided excitatory pulses, 1000 right-sided inhibitory pulses). Treatment led to improvements in clinician-assessed mood ratings, self-report emotional scores (mood, anger, anxiety, and behavioral dyscontrol), fluid cognition, and headaches (Hacker et al., unpublished).

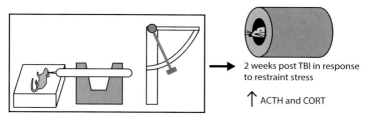

2 weeks post TBI in response to restraint stress

↑ ACTH and CORT

Animal Model of TBI: FPI

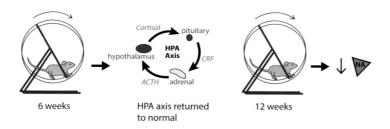

6 weeks

HPA axis returned to normal

12 weeks

FIGURE 4.10.

Recent studies demonstrate that a physical exercise intervention for patients with TBI results in less depressive symptoms, anxiety, and fatigue, as well as improved sleep, community participation, and overall quality of life (Hoffman et al., 2010). Several studies suggest that physical exercise may alleviate depressive symptoms in TBI populations. There is evidence that stress response is heightened for 2 weeks post-mTBI in animal fluid percussion injury (FPI) models (Griesbach et al., 2012). Restraint-induced stress significantly elevated cortisol (CORT) and adrenocorticotrophic hormone (ACTH) levels. Six weeks of daily or intermittent voluntary wheel-running exercise returned the HPA axis to normal stress response for mild stressors (Greisbach et al., 2014). Twelve weeks of 20-min treadmill running resulted in decreased noradrenaline(NA) production during stressful situations.

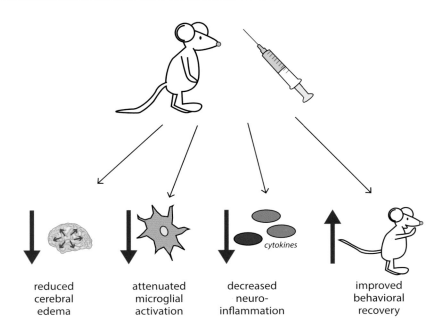

reduced cerebral edema

attenuated microglial activation

decreased neuro-inflammation

cytokines

improved behavioral recovery

FIGURE 4.11.

Methylene blue (MB) has been tested in animals for treatment of depression associated with neuroinflammation. Intravenous MB infusion 15-30 minutes post-TBI reduced cerebral edema, attenuated microglial activation, decreased neuroinflammation, and improved behavioral recovery in TBI mouse model (Talley Watts et al., 2014). Avoid MB if an MAO inhibitor has been administered in the last 14 days; a dangerous drug interaction could occur, leading to serious side effects. There are potential interaction effects with other drugs, thus further testing is needed. Patients with kidney problems should avoid MB treatment (Fenn et al., 2015). Neuroprotective effects may help with neurological recovery from TBI; however, research has been restricted to animals to date, thus clinical trials are needed in humans with TBI.

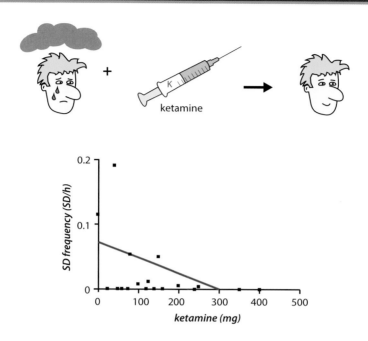

FIGURE 4.12.

Ketamine has been shown to be effective in patients with treatment-resistant depression (TRD) (Frere et al., 2016). Traumatic brain injury (TBI) typically results in elevated levels of glutamate that can persist for several weeks. In contrast to the delayed action of monoamine antidepressant treatment, ketamine exerts rapid and sustained antidepressant effects after a single dose; therefore, it may be an appropriate alternative approach to patients with TBI and TRD. Ketamine's antidepressant effects may be due directly to its NMDA antagonism, or to its downstream stimulation of AMPA receptors, which influence dendritic spine growth (Chang et al., 2013). There is also evidence that ketamine significantly reduces spreading depolarizations in brain-injured patients (Sakowitz et al., 2009). These findings suggest that due to ketamine's neuroprotective effect, this treatment could be particularly beneficial for patients with TBI and TRD; however, additional research is needed.

TRADITIONAL TREATMENT FOR MANIA IN PATIENTS WITH TBI: PHARMACOLOGICAL

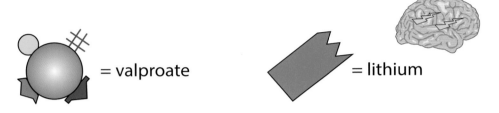

= valproate   = lithium

FIGURE 4.13.

There is limited evidence about specific pharmacotherapy for mania after traumatic brain injury (TBI), however, valproate is recommended as the first-line of treatment. Lithium is recommended as second-line treatment, due to seizure risk (Vaishnavi et al., 2009). Lithium is also known to have neuroprotective properties (Wada et al., 2005), which may be useful for patients recovering from TBI. Additionally, case reports suggest the usefulness of quetiapine, carbamazepine, clonidine, and electroconvulsive therapy (ECT) (Warden et al., 2006; Oster et al., 2007). Isolated psychotherapy is not considered efficient for mania after TBI, although it can be an adjunctive therapy (Schneck, 2002).

TRADITIONAL TREATMENT FOR TBI-RELATED PSYCHOSIS: PHARMACOLOGICAL

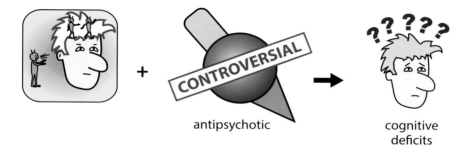

FIGURE 4.14.

The use of antipsychotics in patients with traumatic brain injury (TBI) is controversial because they may further impair cognitive deficits. Typical antipsychotics that have anticholinergic, hypotensive, or sedative effects, or a strong dopaminergic antagonism, may worsen the already existent deficits for TBI survivors. Drugs such as haloperidol could delay the neuronal recuperation (Feeney et al., 1982; Goldstein, 1993), and worsen the patients' prognosis in the short term (Rao et al., 1985). Therefore, atypical antipsychotics are recommended as first-line treatment. The initial doses must be prescribed from one-third to half of the usual ones, increasing them gradually, since patients with TBI-associated psychosis are particularly susceptible to side effects (Arciniegas et al., 2003). Resperidone (Schreiber et al., 1998), as well as respiradone with galantine (Bennouna et al., 2005) have been reported as successfully treating psychosis in this population. Clozadine has also been successful, but the side effects in these patients are adverse (Michals et al., 1993).

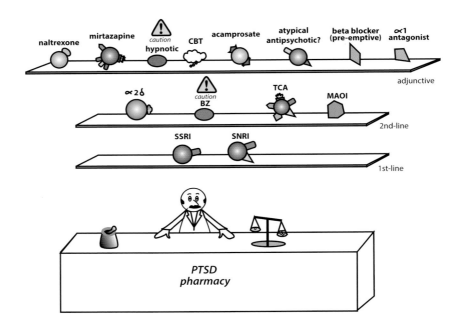

PTSD
pharmacy

FIGURE 4.15.

There are currently no evidence-based guidelines for pharmacologic treatment of Post Traumatic Stress Disorder (PTSD) for patients who have a history of traumatic brain injury (TBI) (Morgan et al., 2012). However, the research encourages using caution with medications that may impair cognition (Kennedy et al., 2007). At this time, it is unknown whether pharmacotherapies used in PTSD are beneficial or safe for patients with comorbid traumatic brain injury (TBI). Useful drugs for PTSD in general, such as antidepressants (especially SSRIs), atypical antipsychotics, and adrenergic blockers are treatment options (Vieweg et al., 2006). The figure captures the first, second, and third line of treatment recommendations for patients with PTSD who do not have TBI, thus caution is recommended. Currently, the only FDA-approved medications for the treatment of PTSD are sertraline and paroxetine. However, paroxetine should be avoided because of its anticholinergic properties, and because this population is particularly sensitive to its adverse side effects. Recent findings suggest that the antipsychotic quetiapine is an effective monotherapy for military-related PTSD. (Villarreal et al., 2016). Future research is needed before specific guidelines can be offered for pharmacological treatment of patients with PTSD and TBI.

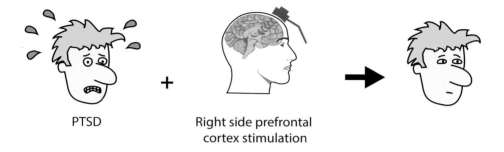

PTSD   Right side prefrontal
              cortex stimulation

FIGURE 4.16.

Pharmacological studies have demonstrated that reduced glutamaterigic neurotransmission, by α-amino-3-hydroxy-5-methyl-4-isoxazolepropionic acid (AMPA) receptor blockage, results in anxiolytic effects, but not all patients respond to pharmacological treatment for PTSD. Studies have shown that administration of low-frequency repetitive transcranial magnetic stimulation (rTMS) on the right dorsolateral prefrontal cortex (DLPFC) is beneficial for improving the symptoms of PTSD (Cohen et al., 2014), in as few as 10 sessions (Garcia-Toro et al., 2002). Neuroimaging studies have shown increased oxygenation of the right prefrontal cortex when participants are exposed to experiences that remind them of traumatic experiences. Low-frequency rTMS (1 Hz) might decrease activity in the cortical areas of the right hemisphere, which may in turn improve abnormalities and reduce cerebral functional asymmetries associated with PTSD (Osuch, et al., 2009) In addition, stimulating the right DLPFC with high frequency pulses activates the hypothalamic-pituitary-adrenal (HPA) axis, inhibiting excessive autonomic response and suppressing activity of the amygdala (Cohen et al., 2004). Thus, both low-frequency and high-frequency, when applied to the right side, are potentially well-suited to reduce symptoms of PTSD.

TRADITIONAL TREATMENT FOR AGGRESSION IN PATIENTS WITH TBI: PHARMACOLOGICAL

Potentially Helpful	Potentially Harmful
Beta blockers (propranolol, pindolol)	Sedating agents
Methylphenidate	Benzodiazepines**
Lithium	Haloperidol
Desipramine	Clonidine
Carbamazepine	
Valproate	
Tricyclic antidepressants	

FIGURE 4.17.

Considering the multifactorial nature of aggression, psychological and social variables that may contribute to this behavior must be approached. The literature about the pharmacotherapy for aggression is wide but with limited evidence strength. The best evidences are available for the betablockers propranolol and pindolol, but other drugs such as tricyclic antidepressants, SSRIs, buspirone, valproic acid, lithium, desipramine, carbamazepine, and methylphenidate have been effective in reducing aggressive symptoms (Warden et al., 2006). Agents that cause sedation or further impair cognition should be avoided if possible. Some evidence suggests that benzodiazepines, haloperidol, and clonidine may impair recovery. Benzodiazepines may be particularly dangerous because they may cause paradoxical agitation in patients with TBI.

SUMMARY

As our understanding of the neurobiological and psychiatric sequelae associated with traumatic brain injury (TBI) expands, it becomes increasingly clear that injury type, severity, and specific brain regions involved may greatly impact the mental health of patients suffering from TBI. Early detection of TBI, along with appropriate diagnosis and timely treatment of associated neuropsychiatric symptoms, is critical. As the state of the research improves, adequately managing high risk populations, and increasing awareness about genetic and environmental risk factors associated with TBI could improve prevention of this devastating, life-altering condition. A variety of biological markers, neuroimaging techniques, and improved neurological/cognitive screening methods could result in earlier detection of TBI, thus allowing for more timely treatment. Pharmacological agents are in development for various neuropsychiatric conditions associated with TBI, and there are many alternative treatment options available that offer potential benefits for patients with TBI.

REFERENCES

Achte K, Jarho L, Kyykka T, Vesterinen E. Paranoid disorders following war brain damage. Preliminary report. Psychopathology 1991;24:309–315.

Ahmed A and Simmons Z. Pseudobulbar affect: prevalence and management. Therapeutics and Clinical Risk Management 2013;9:483-489.

Andersen G, Ingeman-Nielsen M, Vestergaard K, Riis JO. Pathoanatomic correlation between poststroke pathological crying and damage to brain areas involved in serotonergic neurotransmission. Stroke 1994; 25(5):1050–1052.

Anderson V, Catroppa C, Morse S, et al. Recovery of intellectual ability following traumatic brain injury in childhood: impact of injury severity and age at injury. Pediatr Neurosurg 2000;32:282–90.

Araki T, Yokota H, Morita A. Pediatric Traumatic Brain Injury: Characteristic Features, Diagnosis, and Management. Neurologia Medico-Chirurgica 2017;57(2):82-93.

Arciniegas DB, Harris SN, Brousseau KM. Psychosis following traumatic brain injury. Int Rev Psychiatry 2003;15:328–40.

Ayalon L, Borodkin K, Dishon L, Kanety H, Dagan Y. Circadian rhythm sleep disorders following traumatic brain injury. Neurology 2007;68(4):1136-1140.

Barr WB, Prichep LS, Chabot R, Powell MR, McCrea M. Measuring brain electrical activity to track recovery from sport-related concussion. Brain Injury 2012;26(1):58-66.

Barrio JR, Small GW, Wong KP, et al. In vivo characterization of chronic traumatic encephalopathy using [F-18]FDDNP PET brain imaging. PNAS 2015; 112(22): E2039-E2047.

Baumann CR. Traumatic brain injury and disturbed sleep and wakefulness. Neuromolecular Medicine 2012; 14(3): 205-212.

Baumann CR, Werth E, Stocker R, Ludwig S, Bassetti CL. Sleep-wake disturbances 6 months after traumatic brain injury: a prospective study. Brain 2007;130(Pt 7):1873-1883.

Bendlin BB, Makdissi M. Blood-based biomarkers for evaluating sport-related concussion. Neurology 2017 2017;88(6):512-513.

Bennouna M, Greene VB, Defranoux L. Adjuvant galantamine to risperidone improves negative and cognitive symptoms in a patient presenting with schizophrenialike psychosis after traumatic brain injury. J Clin Psychopharmacol 2005;25:505–7.

Bey T, Ostick B. Second Impact Syndrome. The Western Journal of Emergency Medicine 2009;10(1):6-10.

Brain Injury Association of America: www.biausa.org

Brasil-Neto JP, Boechat-Barros R, da Mota-Silveira DA. The use of slow-frequency transcranial magnetic stimulation in the treatment of depression at Brasilia University Hospital: preliminary findings. Arq Neuropsiquiatr 2003;61(1):83-86.

REFERENCES

Broglio SP, Ferrara MS, Macciocchi SN, Baumgartner TA, Elliot R. Test-retest reliability of computerized concussion assessment programs. J Athl Train 2007;42(4):509-514.

Broglio SP, Moore RD, Hillman CH. A history of sport-related concussion on event-related brain potential correlates of cognition. International Journal of Psychophysiology 2011;82(1):16-23.

Brooks BR, Thisted RA, Appel SH, et al. Treatment of pseudobulbar affect in ALS with dextromethorphan/quinidine: a randomized trial. Neurology 2004; 63 (8):1364-70.

Cantu RC. Guidelines for return to contact sports after a cerebral concussion. The Physician and Sports Medicine 1986; 14(10): 75-83.

Cantu RC. Second impact syndrome. Clin Sports Med 1998; 17:37-44.

Casson IR, Viano DC, Haacke EM, Kou Z, LeStrange DG. Is there chronic brain damage in retired NFL players? Neuroradiology, neuropsychology, and neurology examinations of 45 retired players. Sports Health 2014; 6(5): 384-395.

CDC. Traumatic Brain Injury. http://www.cdc.gov/TraumaticBrainInjury/index.html. Accessed January 9, 2012.

Chasle V, Riffaud L, Longuet R, et al. Mild head injury and attention deficit hyperactivity disorder in children. Child's Nervous System 2016;32(12):2357-2361.

Chang LC, Raty SR, Ortiz J, Bailard NS, Mathew SJ. The emerging use of ketamine for anesthesia and sedation in traumatic brain injuries. CNS Neurosci Ther 2013;19(6):390-395.

Chiesa A, Duhaime A-C. Abusive head trauma. Pediatr Clin North Am 2009; 56(2):317–31.

Ciurea AV, Gorgan MR, Tascu A, Sandu AM, Rizea RE. Traumatic brain injury in infants and toddlers, 0-3 years old. Journal of Medicine and Life 2011; 4(3): 234-243.

Cohen H, Kaplan Z, Kotler M, et al. Repetitive transcranial magnetic stimulation of the right dorsolateral prefrontal cortex in posttraumatic stress disorder: a double-blind, placebo-controlled study. Am J Psychiatry 2004; 161(3): 515-524.

Collen J, Orr N, Lettieri CJ, Carter K, Holley AB. Sleep disturbances among soldiers with combat-related traumatic brain injury. Chest 2012; 142(3): 622-630.

Cummings JL, Arciniegas MD, Brooks BR, et al. Defining and Diagnosing Involuntary Emotional Expression Disorder. CNS Spectrums 2006; 11(6): 1-11.

Davison K. Schizophrenia-like psychoses associated with organic cerebral disorders: A review. Psychiatric Developments 1983;1:1–33.

DeKosky ST, Blennow K, Ikonomovic MD, Gandy S. Acute and chronic traumatic encephalopathies: pathogenesis and biomarkers. Nat Rev Neurol 2013;9(4):192-200.

REFERENCES

Diaz AP, Schwarzbold ML, Thais ME, et al. Psychiatric disorders and health-related quality of life after severe traumatic brain injury: a prospective study. Journal of Neurotrauma 2012;29(6):1029-1037.

Eierud C, Nathan DE, Teslovich T. Frontal pole cortical deficits in mild, moderate, and severe traumatic brain injuries. Society for Neuroscience Abstract, 2016, San Diego.

Eslinger PJ, Flaherty-Craig CV, Benton AL. Developmental outcomes after early prefrontal cortex damage. Brain Cogn 2004; 55:84–103.

Ewing-Cobbs L, Prasad MR, Kramer L, et al. Late intellectual and academic outcomes following traumatic brain injury sustained during early childhood. J Neurosurg: Pediatrics 2006;105:287–96.

Fazio VC, Lovell MR, Pardini JE, Collins MW. The relation between post concussion symptoms and neurocognitive performance in concussed athletes. NeuroRehabilitation 2007;22(3):207-216.

Farrer TJ, Frost RB, Hedges DW. Prevalence of traumatic brain injury in intimate partner violence offenders compared to the general population: a meta-analysis. Trauma Violence Abuse 2012; 13(2): 77-82.

Feeney DM, Gonzalez A, Law WA. Amphetamine, haloperidol, and experience interact to affect rate of recovery after motor cortex injury. Science 1982;217:855–7.

Fenn AM, Skendelas JP, Moussa DN, et al. Methylene blue attenuates traumatic brain injury-associated neuroinflammation and acute depressive-like behavior in mice. J Neurotrauma 2015; 32(2): 127-138.

Fichtenberg NL, Zafonte RD, Putnam S, Mann NR, Millard AE. Insomnia in a post-acute brain injury sample. Brain Injury 2002; 16(3): 197-206.

Fletcher, JM, Levin HS, Lachar D, et al. Behavioral outcomes after pediatric closed head injury: Relationships with age, severity, and lesion size. Journal of Child Neurology 1996; 11, 283–290.

Flom L, Fromkin J, Panigrahy A, Tyler-Kabara E, Berger RP. Development of a screening MRI for infants at risk for abusive head trauma. Pediatric Radiology 2015; 4:519-526.

French L, McCrea M, Baggett M. The Military Acute Concussion Evaluation (MACE). Journal of Special Operations Medicine 2008; 8(1): 68-77.

Frencham KA, Fox AM, Mayberry MT. Neuropsychological studies of mild traumatic brain injury: A meta-analytic review of research since 1995. J Clin Exp Neuropsychol 2005; 27:334–351.

Frere M, and Tepper J. Ketamine: future treatment for unresponsive depression? Irish Medicine Journal 2016; 109(8): 453.

REFERENCES

Fujii DE, Ahmed I. Risk factors in psychosis secondary to traumatic brain injury. Journal of Neuropsychiatry Clinics in Neuroscience 2001;13:61–69.

Garcia-Toro M, Saliva Coll J, Crespi' Font M, et al. Panic disorder and transcranial magnetic stimulation. Actas Esp Psiquiatr 2002; 30(4): 221-224.

Golding EM, Robertson CS, Bryan RM. The consequences of traumatic brain injury on cerebral blood flow and autoregulation: a review. Clinical and Experimental Hypertension 1999; 21(4): 299-332.

Goldstein LB. Basic and clinical studies of pharmacologic effects on recovery from brain injury. J Neural Transplant Plast 1993;4:175–92.

Goldsmith W, Plunkett. A biomechanical analysis of the causes of traumatic brain injury in infants and children. Am J Forensic Med Pathol 2004; 25: 89–100.

Gosselin N, Lassonde M, Petit D et al. Sleep following sport-related concussions. Sleep Med 2009; 10, 35–46.

Griesbach GS, Tio DL, Nair S, Novda DA. Recovery of stress response coincides with responsiveness to voluntary exercise after traumatic brain injury. J Neurotrauma 2014; 31(7): 674-682.

Hillbom E. After-effects of brain-injuries. Research on the symptoms causing invalidism of persons in finland having sustained brain-injuries during the wars of 1939–1940 and 1941–1944. Acta Psychiatrica Supplement 1960;35:1–195.

Hoffer ME, Balaban C, Slade MD, Tsao JW, Hoffer B. Amelioration of acute sequelae of blast induced mild traumatic brain injury by N-acetyl cysteine: a double-blind, placebo controlled study. PLOS One 2013; 8(1): 1-10.

Hoffman JM, Bell KR, Powell JM, et al. A randomized controlled trial of exercise to improve mood after traumatic brain injury. PMR 2010; 2(10): 911-919.

Hoofien D, Gilboa A, Vakil E, Donovick PJ. Traumatic brain injury (TBI) 10–20 years later: A comprehensive outcome study of psychiatric symptomatology, cognitive abilities and psychosocial functioning. Brain Injury 2001; 15:189–209.

Iannone A, Cruz AP, Brasil-Neto JP, Boechat-Barros R. Transcranial magnetic stimulation and transcranial direct current stimulation appear to be safe neuromodulatory techniques useful in the treatment of anxiety disorders and other neuropsychiatric disorders. Arq Neuropsiquiatr 2016; 74(10): 829-835.

Iverson, KM, Dardis, CM, Pogoda, TK. Traumatic brain injury and PTSD symptoms as a consequence of intimate partner violence. Comprehensive Psychiatry 2017; 74:80-87.

Jotwani V, Harmon KG. Postconcussion syndrome in athletes. Curr Sports Med Rep 2010;9(1):21-26.

REFERENCES

Kemp S, Biswas R, Neumann V, Coughlan A. The value of melatonin for sleep disorders occurring post-head injury: a pilot RCT. Brain Injury 2004; 18(9): 911-919.

Kennedy JE, Jaffee MS, Leskin GA, et al. Posttraumatic stress disorder and posttraumatic stress disorder-like symptoms and mild traumatic brain injury. Journal of Rehabilitation Research and Development 2007; 44:895-920.

Kim PT, Falcone RA. Nonaccidental trauma in pediatric surgery. The Surgical Clinics North America 2017; 97(1): 21-33.

Kim SW, Shin IS, Kim JM, Lim SY, et al. Mirtazapine treatment for pathological laughing and crying after stroke. Clin. Neuropharmacol 2005; 28(5), 249-251.

Koerte IK, Hufschmidt J, Muehlmann M, Lin AP, Shenton ME. Advanced neuroimaging of mild traumatic brain injury. Translational Research in Traumatic Brain Injury 2016; Chapter 13.

Kraus N, Thompson EC, Krizman J, et al. Auditory biological marker of concussion in children. Scientific Reports 2016; 6: 1-10.

Kraus MF, Susmaras T, Caughlin BP, et al. White matter integrity and cognition in chronic traumatic brain injury: a diffusion tensor imaging study. Brain 2007;130 (Pt 10):2508-2519.

Langlois JA, Rutland-Brown W, Wald MM. The epidemiology and impact of traumatic brain injury: a brief overview. J Head Trauma Rehabil 2006;21(5):375-378.

Larson EB, and Zollman FS. The effect of sleep medications on cognitive recovery from traumatic brain injury. The Journal of Head Trauma Rehabilitation 2010; 25(1): 61-67.

Lee JS, Han MK, Kim SH, Kwon OK, Kim JH. Fiber tracking by diffusion tensor imaging in corticospinal tract stroke: topographical correlation with clinical symptoms. Neuroimage 2005; 26(3): 771-776.

Letson MM, Cooper JN, Deans KJ, et al. Prior opportunities to identify abuse in children with abusive head trauma. Child Abuse and Neglect 2016; 60: 36-45.

Levin HS, and Chapman SB. Aphasia after TBI. In: Sarno MT, ed. Acquired Aphasia. 3rd ed. San Diego, CA: Academic Press. 1998;481-529.

Levin, H. S., Goldstein, F. C., Williams, D. H., & Eisenberg, H. M. The contribution of frontal lobe lesions to the neurobehavioral outcome in closed head injury. In Levin HS & Eisenberg HM, Benton AI, eds. Frontal Lobe Function and Dysfunction (pp. 318–338). New York: Oxford University Press; 1991.

Levin HS, Culhane KA, Mendelsohn D, et al. Cognition in relation to magnetic resonance imaging in head-injured children and adolescents. Arch Neurol 1993; 50:897–905.

Leung A, Shukla S, Fallah A, et al. Repetitive transcranial magnetic stimulation in managing mild traumatic brain injury-related headaches. Neuromodulation 2016; 19(2): 133-141.

REFERENCES

MacMillan HL, Wathen N, Jamieson E. Screening for intimate partner violence in health care settings: a randomized trial. JAMA 2009; 302(5): 493-501.

Magnuson J, Leonessa F, Ling GS. Neuropathology of explosive blast traumatic brain injury. Current Neurology and Neuroscience Reports 2012; 12(5): 570-579.

Maroon J, Lovell MR, Norwig J et al. Cerebral concussion in athletes: evaluation and neuropsychological testing. Neurosurgery. 2000; 47:659-669.

Masel BE, Scheibel RS, Kimbark T, Kuna ST. Excessive daytime sleepiness in adults with brain injuries. Archives of Physical Medicine and Rehabilitation 2001; 82(11): 1526-1532.

Maurice T, Urani A, Phan VL, Romieu P. The interaction between neuroactive steroids and 6-1 receptor function: behavioral consequences and therapeutic opportunities. Brain Res. Rev 2001; 37(1–3), 116–132.

Max JE, Levin HS, Schachar RJ, et al. Predictors of personality change due to traumatic brain injury in children and adolescents six to twenty-four months after injury. J Neuropsychiatry Clin Neurosci 2006; 18:21–32.

McAllister TW. Neurobiological consequences of traumatic brain injury. Dialogues in Clinical Neuroscience 2011; 13(3): 288-300.

McCrea M, Prichep L, Powell MR, Chabot R, Barr WB. Acute effects and recovery after sport-related concussion: a neurocognitive and quantitative brain electrical activity study. Journal of Head Trauma Rehabilitation 2010; 25(4): 283-292.

McKee AC, Cantu, RC, Nowinski, CJ, et al. Chronic traumatic encephalopathy in athletes: progressive tauopathy after repetitive head injury. Journal of Neuropathology and Experimental Neurology 2009; 68(7): 709-735.

McKee AC, Stern, RA, Nowinski CJ, et al. The spectrum of disease in chronic traumatic encephalopathy. Brain 2013; 136(Pt 1): 43-64.

McKenna PJ, Kane JM, Parrish K. Psychotic syndromes in epilepsy. American Journal of Psychiatry 1985; 142:895–904.

McLendon LA, Kralik SF, Grayson PA, Golomb MR. The controversial second impact syndrome: a review of the literature. Pediatric Neurology 2016; 62:9-17.

Michael AP, Stout J, Roskos PT, et al. Evaluation of Cortical Thickness after Thickness after Traumatic Brain Injury in Military Veterans. Journal of Neurotrauma 2015; 32(22); 1751-1758.

Michals ML, Crismon ML, Roberts S, et al. Clozapine response and adverse effects in nine brain-injured patients. J Clin Psychopharmacol 1993;13:198–203.

Miller A, Pratt H, Schiffer RB. Pseudobulbar affect: the spectrum of clinical presentations, etiologies and treatments. Expert Review of Neurotherapeutics 2011; 11(7): 1077-1088.

REFERENCES

Molloy C, Conroy RM, Cotter DR, Cannon M. Is traumatic brain injury a risk factor for schizophrenia? A meta-analysis of case-controlled population-based studies. Schizophrenia Bulletin 2011; 37(6): 1104-1110.

Morgan M, Lockwood A, Steinke D, Schleenbaker R, Botts, S. Pharmacotherapy regimens among patients with posttraumatic stress disorder and mild traumatic brain injury. Psychiatric Services 2012; 63(2): 182-185.

Murray CE, Lundgren K, Olson LN, Hunnicutt G. Practice update: what professionals who are not brain injury specialists need to know about intimate partner violence-related traumatic brain injury. Trauma Violence Abuse 2016: 17(3): 298-305.

Okie S. Traumatic brain injury in the war zone. N Engl J Med 2005;352(20):2043-2047.

Oster TJ, Anderson CA, Filley CM, et al. Quetiapine for mania due to traumatic brain injury. CNS Spectr. 2007;12:764–9.

Osuch EA, Benson BE, Luckenbaugh DA, et al. Repetitive TMS combined with exposure therapy for PTSD: a preliminary study. J Anxiety Disord 2009; 23(1): 54-59.

Panitch HS, Thisted RA, Smith RA et al. Randomized, controlled trial of dextromethorphan/quinidine for pseudobulbar affect in multiple sclerosis. Ann. Neurol 2006; 59(5): 780–787.

Paranjape A, Rask K, Liebschutz J. Utility of STaT for the identification of recent intimate partner violence. Journal of the National Medical Association 2006; 98(10): 1663-1669.

Parks SE, Kegler SR, Annest JL, et al. Characteristics of fatal abusive head trauma among children in the USA, 2003-2007: an application of the CDC operational case definition to national vital statistics data. Inj Prev 2011;18(3):193–9.

Parvizi J, Arciniegas DB, Bernardini GL, et al. Diagnosis and management of pathological laugher and crying. Mayo Clinic Proceedings 2006; 81(11): 1482-1486.

Peskind ER, Petrie EC, Cross DJ, et al. Cerebrocerebellar hypometabolism associated with repetitive blast exposure mild traumatic brain injury in 12 Iraq war Veterans with persistent post-concussive symptoms. Neuroimage. 2011; 54(suppl 1): S76-S82.

Picard RG. How violence is justified: sinn fein's an phoblacht. Journal of Communication 1991; 41(4): 90-103.

Prigatano GP, Gale SD. The current status of postconcussion syndrome. Curr Opin Psychiatry 2011;24(3):243-250.

Prichep LS, McCrea M, Barr W, Powell M, Chabot RJ. Time course of clinical and electrophysiological recovery after sport-related concussion. The Journal of Head Trauma Rehabilitation 2013; 28(4): 266-273.

Poeck K. Pathological laughing and weeping in patients with progressive balbar palsy. German Medical Monthly 1969; 14(8): 394-397.

REFERENCES

Pope Jr. HG, McElroy SL, Satlin A, et al. Head injury, bipolar disorder and response to valproate. Compr Psychiatry 1988; 29:34–38.

Pope LE, Khalil MH, Berg JE, et al. Pharmacokinetics of dextromethorphan after single or multiple dosing in combination with quinidine in extensive and poor metabolizers. J. Clin. Pharmacol 2004; 44(10): 1132–1142.

Rao N, Jellinek HM, Woolston DC. Agitation in closed head injury: haloperidol effects on rehabilitation outcome. Arch Phys Med Rehabil 1985;66:30–4.

Resch J, Driscoll A, McCaffrey N, et al. ImPact Test-Retest Reliabilty: Reliably Unreliable? J Athl Train 2013; 48(4): 506-511.

Rogers JM, Read CA. Psychiatric comorbidity following traumatic brain injury. Brain Injury 2009; 21(13-14): 1321-1333.

Rice VJ, Lindsay G, Overby C, et al. Automated Neuropsychological Metrics (ANAM) Traumatic Brain Injury (TBI): Human Factors Assessment. Army Research Laboratory 2011; 1-42.

Sachdev P, Smith JS, Cathcart S. Schizophrenia-like psychosis following traumatic brain injury: A chart-based descriptive and case-control study. Psychological Medicine 2001; 31:231–239.

Sakowitz OW, Kiening KL, Krajewski KL, et al. Preliminary evidence that ketamine inhibits spreading depolarizations in acute human brain injury. Stroke 2009; 40(8): e519-22.

Sayer NA. Traumatic brain injury and its neuropsychiatric sequelae in war veterans. Annual Review of Medicine 2012; 63: 405-419.

Saunders R, Harbaugh R. The second impact in catastrophic contact sports head trauma. JAMA 1984; 252:538-539.

Schneck CD. Bipolar disorder in neurologic illness. Curr Treat Options Neurol 2002;4:477–86.

Schreiber S, Klag E, Gross Y, et al. Beneficial effect of risperidone on sleep disturbance and psychosis following traumatic brain injury. Int Clin Psychopharmacol 1998;13:273–5.

Seliger GM, Hornstein A, Flax J, Herbert J, Schroeder K. Fluoxetine improves emotional incontinence. Brain Injury 1992; 6(3): 267-270.

Serafini G, Howland RH, Rovedi F, Girardi P, Amore M. The role of ketamine in treatment-resistant depression: a systematic review. Curr Neuropharmacol 2014; 12(5): 444-461.

Sherin KM, Sinacore JM, Li XQ, Zitter RE, Shakil A. HITS: A short domestic violence screening tool for use in a family practice setting. Family Medicine 1998; 30(7): 508-511.

Silver JM, McAllister TW, Arciniegas DB. Depression and cognition complaints following mild traumatic brain injury. Am J Psychiatry 2009; 166(6): 653-661.

REFERENCES

Silver JM, Kramer R, Greenwald S, Weissman M. The association between head injuries and psychiatric disorders: Findings from the New Haven NIMH Epidemiologic Catchment Area Study. Brain Injury 2001;15:935–945.

Silverberg N, Iverson G. Etiology of the post-concussion syndrome: physiogenesis and psychogensis revisited . Neurorehabilitation 2011; 29: 317-329.

Siman R, Giovannone N, Hanten G, et al. Evidence that the blood biomarker SNTF predicts brain imaging changes and persistent cognitive dysfunction in mild TBI patients. Frontiers in Neurobiology 2013; 4(190): 1-8.

Sohal H, Eldridge S, Feder G. The sensitivity and specificity of four questions (HARK) to identify intimate partner violence: a diagnostic accuracy study in general practice. BMC Fam Pract 2007; 8(49): 1-9.

Starkstein SE, Pearlson GD, Boston J, et al. Mania after brain injury: a controlled study of causative factors. Arch Neurol 1987; 44:1069–1073.

Stuss DT, Benson DF. The frontal lobes and control of cognition and memory. In E. Perecman (Ed.), The Frontal Lobes Revisited (pp. 141–158). New York: The IRBN Press; 1987.

Talley Watts L, Long JA, Chemello J. Methylene blue is neuroprotective against mild traumatic brain injury. J Neurotrauma 2014; 31 (11): 1063-1071.

Teasdale G, Jennett, B. Assessment of coma and impaired consciousness. A practical scale. Lancet 1974; 2(7872): 81-84.

Vaishnavi S, Rao V, Fann JR. Neuropsychiatric problems after traumatic brain injury: unraveling the silent epidemic Psychosomatics 2009; 50(3): 198-205.

van Reekum R, Cohen T, Wong J. Can traumatic brain injury cause psychiatric disorders? Journal of Neuropsychiatry and Clinical Neurosciences. 2000;12(3):316-327.

Varney NR, Menefee L. Psychosocial and executive deficits following closed head injury: Implications for orbital frontal cortex. Journal of Head Trauma Rehabilitation. 1993;8:32–44.

Vieweg WV, Julius DA, Fernandez A, et al. Posttraumatic stress disorder: clinical features, pathophysiology, and treatment. Am J Med 2006;119:383–90.

Villarreal G, Hamner ME, Canive JM, et al. Efficacy of quetiapine monotherapy in posttraumatic stress disorder: a randomized, placebo-controlled trial. Am J Psychiatry 2016; 173(12): 1205-1212.

Wada A, Yokoo H, Yanagita T, et al. Lithium: potential therapeutics against acute brain injuries and chronic neurodegenerative diseases. J Pharmacol Sci. 2005;99:307–21.

Walker KR, Tesco G. Molecular mechanisms of cognitive dysfunction following traumatic brain injury. Frontiers Aging Neurosci Rev 2013;5(29):1-25.

REFERENCES

Warden DL, Gordon B, McAllister TW, et al. Guidelines for the pharmacologic treatment of neurobehavioral sequelae of traumatic brain injury. J Neurotrauma 2006; 23(10): 1468-1501.

Weiss SJ, Ernst AA, Cham E, Nick TG. Development of a screen for ongoing intimate partner violence. Violence Vict 2003; 18(2): 131-141.

Werling LL, Keller A, Frank JG, Nuwayhid SJ. A comparison of the binding profiles of dextromethorphan, memantine, fluoxetine and amitriptyline: treatment of involuntary emotional expression disorder. Exp. Neurol 2007; 207(2): 248–257.

Wilde EA, McCauley SR, Hunter JV, et al. Diffusion tensor imaging of acute mild traumatic brain injury in adolescents. Neurology 2008; 70(12): 948-955.

Wortzel HS, and Arciniegas DB. Treatment of post-traumatic cognitive impairments. Curr Treat Options Neurol 2012; 14(5): 493-508.

Wu H, Shao A, Zhao M, et al. Melatonin attenuates neuronal apoptosis through up-regulation of K (+) -Cl(-) cotransporter KCC2 expression following traumatic brain injury in rats. J Pineal Res 2016; 61(2):1-10.

Ylvisaker M, Feeney T, Szekeres F. Social-environmental approach to communication and behavior. In M. Ylvisaker (Ed.), Traumatic Brain Injury Rehabilitation: Children and Adolescents (2nd ed., pp. 271–302). Boston: Butterworth-Heinemann; 1998

Zappalà G, Thiebaut de Schotten M, Eslinger PJ. Traumatic brain injury and the frontal lobes: what can we gain with diffusion tensor imaging? Cortex 2012; 48(2):156-65.

Zetterberg H, Smith DH, Kaj B. Biomarkers of mild traumatic brain injury in cerebrospinal fluid and blood. Nature Reviews Neurology 2013; 9: 201-210.

Zhdanova IV, Wurtman RJ, Regan MM, et al. Melatonin treatment for age-related insomnia. J Clin Endocrinol Metab 2001; 86(10):4727-4730.

OPTIONAL POSTTEST AND CME CERTIFICATE

Release / CME Expiration Dates

Print Monograph Released: August, 2017

Electronic Books Released: August, 2017

CME Credit Expires: August, 2020

Posttest Study Guide

The posttest questions have been provided below solely as a study tool to prepare for your online submission. **NOTE: Posttests can only be submitted online. Faxed/mailed copies of the posttest cannot be processed** and will be returned to the sender.

1. Chris is a 28-year old marine on active duty. He has been complaining of dizziness, extreme headaches, and memory problems related to traumatic brain injury. His neurological injuries are most likely the effect of:

   A. Direct blunt trauma, resulting in damage to underlying tissues

   B. Diffuse axonal damage as the result of a blast-induced injury

   C. Rotational acceleration/deceleration, resulting in focal and diffuse trauma

2. Robert is a 31-year old professional football player who has been feeling apathetic, and has experienced severe memory problems, and impaired judgment. His PET scans reveal tau deposits in the periaqueductal gray (PAG) in the dorsal midbrain (A and B) and in amygdala. The patient is most likely suffering from:

   A. Second Impact Syndrome (SIS)

   B. Abusive Head Trauma (AHT)

   C. Chronic Traumatic Encephalopathy (CTE)

3. Maria is a 22-year old woman who has been complaining of headaches, dizziness, and memory problems. In addition, there are bruises on her neck and arms. She mentions that she is in an intimate relationship with someone who has a bad temper. What is NOT an appropriate approach for the screening of traumatic brain injury in this patient?

   A. Immediate Post-Concussive Assessment and Cognitive Testing (ImPACT) alone is a sufficient screening tool

   B. Acute Concussion Evaluation (ACE) and Hurt, Insult, Threaten, Scream (HITS)

   C. ImPACT and Slapped, Threatened, and Throw (STaT)

4. Damage to which brain region, as a result of traumatic brain injury, is most associated with apathy?

   A. Dorsolateral prefrontal cortex

   B. Anterior cingulate cortex

   C. Hippocampus

   D. Inferolateral prefrontal cortex

5. Sara, who is 8 months old, was recently diagnosed with abusive head trauma (AHT) after being admitted to the emergency room (ER). She had been seen by her pediatrician several times before, and there were prior opportunities to detect AHT. According to the most current research findings, which of the following prior opportunities is most associated with AHT?

   A. Contact with Child Protective Services (CPS)

   B. Bruising on the infant

   C. Vomiting

6. Which of the following is NOT an overlapping symptom of Post Traumatic Stress Disorder (PTSD) and Persistent Post Concussive Syndrome (PPCS):

   A. Depression/Anxiety

   B. Dizziness

   C. Insomnia

   D. Irritability/Anger

7. Mark recently suffered a combat-related blunt force traumatic brain injury (TBI), and since then has experienced severe sleep disruption. According to recent published findings, which of the following types of sleep disturbances is Mark likely experiencing?

   A. Insomnia

   B. Hypersomnia

   C. Obstructive Sleep Apnea

8. Which of the following general guidelines is NOT recommended for treatment of a patient with traumatic brain injury (TBI):

   A. Hold sessions in a dim lighted room because they could be light sensitive

   B. Speak quickly so that the patient will be motivated to stay on pace

   C. Encourage the patient to keep a written notebook of notes from each session

   D. Allow extra time for patient arrival

OPTIONAL POSTTEST AND CME CERTIFICATE

9. Amanda is a treatment-resistant patient with traumatic brain injury (TBI) and Major Depressive Disorder (MDD). Repetitive transcranial magnetic stimulation (rTMS) may help alleviate Amanda's depressive symptoms by:

   A. Applying low-frequency stimulation to the right dorsolateral prefrontal cortex

   B. Applying low-frequency stimulation to the right ventromedial prefrontal cortex

   C. Applying high frequency stimulation to the left dorsolateral prefrontal cortex

   D. A and C

10. Which type of medication may be particularly dangerous when treating aggression in patients with traumatic brain injury (TBI) because it could cause paradoxical agitation?

    A. Benzodiazepines

    B. Haloperidol

    C. Clonodine

    D. Propranolol

11. I commit to making the following change(s) in my practice as a result of participating in this activity.

    A. Screen for traumatic brain injury in my practice

    B. Screen for neuropsychiatric symptoms associated with traumatic brain injury

    C. A and B

    D. I am already doing both of the above

OPTIONAL POSTTEST AND CME CERTIFICATE

Instructions for Optional Posttest and CME Certificate

There is no posttest fee nor fee for CME credits.

1. Read the book
2. Complete the posttest only online at www.neiglobal.com/CME (under "Book")
3. Print your certificate (if a score of 70% or more is achieved)

Questions? call 888-535-5600, or email
CustomerService@NEIglobal.com